AN IMPOSSIBLE WOMAN

The Memories of
Dottoressa Moor of Capri

Edited and with an Epilogue by

Graham Greene

THE VIKING PRESS NEW YORK

Published in 1976 by The Viking Press, Inc.
625 Madison Avenue, New York, N.Y. 10022

SBN 670-39421-1
Library of Congress catalog card number:
75-42796

Printed in U.S.A.

'Darling Dottoressa, you are hopeless.'
'Please?'
'Hopeless. Crazy.'
'Crazy, yes, you tell me a truth. But this
with me is no new affair. What I must do I
must do. You are right, I am a wild one.
So I am, so let me be.'

A conversation with
Kenneth Macpherson in Capri, 1951

EDITOR'S NOTE

The preparation of this book for publication owes more than I can explain to Kenneth Macpherson who was working on it when he died. If he had been able to finish what he had begun, it would have been so much the better book.

Perhaps a few words may be said about the editing. Dottoressa Moor was 'interviewed' by someone who had not previously known her (Kenneth and I suggested the main questions he should ask). Her words were recorded—in German—on tape. The result was then translated literally into English for this edition, but I wanted to reproduce, if it was possible, the tone of her voice, so unmistakably her own. She had often recounted these adventures and experiences to me in the years after I had first met her in 1948, in her vivid and incorrect English. A smooth grammatical translation would have been treachery.

Kenneth Macpherson, who had known her as Norman Douglas's doctor on Capri for longer than I had, undertook at my request the task of 'translating the translation'. I have tried to pick up where death stopped him in mid-course—I have even stolen the first seven lines of the introduction he failed to finish. Nor have I hesitated on occasion to insert memories which did not appear on the tapes because the right question was not asked.

Graham Greene

CONTENTS

Part 3

Part 4

Epilogue
by Graham Greene

PREFACE

It is the eyes you do not forget. They are blue. They would do for Chartres.

Their colour changes as weather and times of day change. When they are grey, as the sky and sea of Capri are sometimes grey, all at once a blade of light slashes their idleness into action. The stubborn sulk of the weather lifts and there is a blaze of life. The grey weight was only in the seasoned bones, the old heavy body, in which lies hidden the young girl who wanted to be a nun, the young woman with her uncountable lovers (even the names get confused sometimes in her head). Young? Yes, though she was nearly seventy when her last affair was broken.

More even than the words of her recall, the eyes recite the wild and frightful epic. The laughter and the self-pity are mingled. We must be patient with the self-pity. There was a great deal to pity, and pity cannot always be found in others, and the laughter nearly always returns when she remembers . . . especially when she remembers her lovers.

At seventy-seven years old the Dottoressa speaks. It is January 1962; she is on a brief holiday from Anacapri where she can no longer practise her medicine, and she confides in her friend, Kenneth Macpherson, who shares many of her memories, though he cannot recall so far a past. No one can. She has survived nearly everyone, and she is going to go on surviving—first her best-loved younger son, Andrea, born 'under the rose'; her eldest son Ludovico is soon to die; her beloved grandson, the little Andrea, has been electrocuted under her eyes in a Zurich shoeshop, her friends, Norman Douglas, Compton Mackenzie, Cecil Gray (ghosts of the old Capri), the enemies who had stoned her in the streets of Anacapri when she came there to serve the poor, the doctors who had plotted against her from jealousy—all have gone. Sometimes she regrets even her enemies. Hate as well as love has given salt to her strange disordered life.

'It was a lovely time, this time of pain, compared with now, when I am so very discontented with myself. It is, you see, because no longer do I have a fulfilling occupation and no real longing.

'Do not improve me; for me this is abominable, too; not any more to run everywhere to help those poor ones in Capri who were ill and so afraid because they did not understand.

'No more can I remain in a household being idle where always they are dissatisfied with me, because in these difficult days I myself become difficult.

'This suffering is because all I ever did was run to the people, yes, to the poor ones, and sometimes they gave me fish in return, or fruit or what they had, and this I ate among them. Yes, this was a happiness.

'Now I am too afraid that I will do something wrong. What a big swindle it is to say that we need a companion to talk to. When we are together, there is only dispute or silence. The silence I can do better alone and the dispute makes me too unhappy. And so, you see, it is in this way, yes.

'They tell me I dispute. Yes. But this is in another

way. My dispute is not this narrow one. Too much I have loved my life among people and understood why I must dispute with them and for them and because of what they must endure. This is a big matter. To be a little bit useful is to put a sail on your boat. So fast you can get along and all is right.

'So now I tell you that the people to whom I gave a lot as doctor as well as a person now give me almost nothing at all.

'My very own children, on whom I had pinned all my hopes for my old age, cannot come up to the expectations I had. It never becomes a warm being-together. Why do I only want happiness with others, and why am I not now self-sufficient?

'Even now, in the warm room with such fine music on the wireless, my wishes reach out to be with my children, my friends. But when I am with them, in a short time I long to be back in my solitude.

'Real satisfaction I can find only in nature, music, a lecture or a book, but instead of giving myself up completely to these satisfactions, I am again drawn to people. Too much have I lived with them and for them, and hence being alone is so difficult although it is the most beautiful. What a very dissatisfied person I am, to the roots of my being!

'Even if the shock gets less the pain gets bigger, and only great fatigue can ease it a little. That's why I run around all the time.

'I can feel it like being quite lost that no longer do people matter to me. I mustn't think of the future, and must only live in the past, but these thoughts, these memories hurt too much. Why go further? Without anyone to love deeply, I can't live, but if I find someone to love, then fate will snatch him away again. So where am I to find the courage?

'Can't I be like other people? They take pleasure in each other and in many things, and don't concentrate everything on one *person*. Yes; I loved my big Andrea and then my little Andrea *too* well. Only *they* meant anything to me. Only *they* gave pure happiness, pure joy. Twice God took my most dear ones, both in a terrible way, and what does He give me in return? Only more pain . . .

'Oh, please fetch me, what more can You have in store for me?'

If the friend to whom she was speaking had been a prophet, he would have said, 'A great many years, Dottoressa, and much more pain. I shall die long before you.' To grow very old is to enter the region of death without dying. Only when she is asked to remember old comedies and old loves, the blue eyes light up with sexual joy and her laugh cracks out, like a stone breaking. Memories are her refuge from loneliness.

Graham Greene

PART

1

The Hairdressers' Child

You want to know all that has happened to me. From the beginning? So far back as that. *Santa Madonna*!

I may talk as I want? Good, good, this is good, if I must talk at all. Because for me there is not a beginning or a middle or yet an end. So with a picture you do not start to see it in one corner, but must experience the whole of it first, *then* the examination.

My father was a hairdresser and my mother also a hairdresser, to the Court. She visited the ladies, all those titled ladies who must attend the Empress, and she dressed hair.

Every morning she had to curl them and do what you must do with hair.

Father had a shop in Vienna in the Stephansplatz, just on the corner of the Singerstrasse, and I was a child thrown onto my own resources. But a child does not yet experience loneliness, because of these resources. My father was in the shop each morning, and my mother went off dressing hair and I was alone. Alone in the flat.

As I remember, Mama told me once that she found me on the floor with the cat and that I lapped milk with the cat. But I cannot make such a spoon of the end of my tongue as does a cat. Yes, he was a fat cat, but he was no more a he, poor him.

And that flat, Number 9 on the Neuer Markt, was a large house and perhaps it still stands. And we were in the furthest courtyard at the back. The third courtyard. And there we had these rooms with barred windows.

And, not to be too much a prisoner, I hung my feet out of them and called to people to admire my new shoes . . . and '*Ja!*' they called up to me. 'You are a lucky child. Such fine new shoes.'

Why did I have to say *new shoes*? Forgive me, I cannot go on. Give me one little moment . . .

With my little Andrea, my grandson, it was also a matter of new shoes. They had scratched the shiny soles in order that he should not slide and fall. Such good strong shoes, he was at once so proud of them and indifferent too, and I was at the cash-desk paying for these shoes to the cashier in the shoeshop in Zurich. He had them on his feet, yes, he was wearing them. To walk out into the Bahnhofstrasse in Zurich. But first he had to see how his toes looked in one of those X-ray machines they had in all the shoeshops. So smart they thought them those machines. You will find them no more, but first my little Andrea had to die. My daughter cried, 'Help him! Help him!' But when I turned my little Andrea was already dead. Yes, there, in that shoeshop. Dead, electrocuted . . . My daughter cried, 'You are a doctor. Help him.' But a doctor cannot help the dead.

Turn off this damn machine you make me speak to. Too much I have made myself suffer. I must pace in the room. You will excuse; we wait a little, yes? So . . .

Always Alone

In the Singerstrasse there is Papa's hair-shop. It was a lovely hairdressing salon on the first floor, with a separate entrance on the ground floor. Very lovely it was. Beautiful mirrors, very light, and he had a good, a very good Viennese clientèle. Yes, and then the flat was transferred from Neuer Markt Number 9 to Singer-strasse, and then there I was as a child. Mama went hairdressing as before, and again I was alone in the room. Yes, that fat cat was still there.

No servants, no. Nobody. Always quite alone. That is why I perpetrated several things. For instance, I cut up picture books into a large heap and then set fire to it.

But you must understand that this was not wicked, it was a big adventure of the imagination. It was nearly a disaster too, and Mama was very cross, because she said one of the apprentices who hairdressed could have looked in on me. But nobody ever bothered to look in on me.

Another time, I got hold of the rat-poison and nearly poisoned myself. If a child is left so alone, as they left me alone, these things happen.

But I have lovely memories too. There were the pigeons, so many pigeons who came to the windows and I fed them. No, no, not with rat-poison, this stuff no more I wished to see. I fed them with bread. There was a whetstone to sharpen the razors and I liked to turn it and get hold of the knives to cut the bread and of course I cut myself. Yes, a deep cut. Always, you see, from the beginning, there were accidents. These were small accidents. It was later came the big ones.

That was a lovely time, and most lovely it was that from there I could see the Corpus Christi procession so well. It was the last in which the Empress walked, because later she never walked in it. There was the whole Court. The Emperor's and that of the Empress; all those ladies with all their hair crimped by Mama. It was not the Empress Zita, it was the Empress Elizabeth, and she was a *magnifique* woman, and the Emperor he was Franz Josef. This was in 1888. I was three or four years old. That's when this lovely Corpus Christi procession happened.

In later years I sat, of course, grandly at the cash-desk and took notice like a governor of a bank. With Mama always away dressing all the hair of the Court ladies, it was a way of life. So as not to be any more quite alone and burning the picture books and cutting my hands and drinking rat-poison, I sat there. Yes, and sometimes the cat was there, too, asleep. He was a good cat. Behind the cash-register, yes. No more did I lap milk.

My parents had come from Germany. Both of them. Papa, he was from the Rhine, and Mama from near Stuttgart. And in Vienna, in Saint Stephan's Church, was the marriage. They came to Vienna because two great-uncles lived there. One was Josef Lauber, the Vice-Mayor of Vienna, and the other one was Peter Lehr, who was a gynaecologist, which for those days was to be very renowned. He had a lot to do. You may imagine how it was. And so my parents came to Vienna to help those great-uncles, because Josef Lauber was paralysed on one side. Vice-Mayor he had been, but at this time already he was an old gentleman. And Peter Lehr, he still went on visits; they had their own carriage and horses, and a landau and a 'Brummer' growler. The horses' names were Bubi and Gigerl, two greys and these he drove.

That was in the Einsiedlergasse. And there they had their house. And from there he drove on his professional visits by day and night with his carriage and horses. They had a coachman too. The coachman was at the same time the *concierge* of the house.

20

It was a three-storey house. It still stands. In the Fifth District, with a lovely back courtyard with two pear trees. I romped about there. I collected the horse-droppings in the wheelbarrow from the whole Einsiedlergasse and chucked them on to the dungheap in the back yard, although the dungheap was full from our own stables. I wrestled there with the children. I could never be a respectable girl.

Nearly every day in that part of the world there was a corpse. There happened then the galloping consumption and there were funerals every day. And in the three-storey house in which we lived I went to one. The band came into the entrance of the house and played, and then they carried the dead one out. He was not one of the household, but it had happened in the house. It made a big impression on me. So I ran then (what a pity for my parents who grieved for my behaviour) to all the funerals. I ran behind with the music. They blew into all this brass until they were red and puffed out like faces of Breughel people. Always music attracted me, and when later I studied in High School and there was this castle band, I ran wild. The impulse was more strong than I; this running wild. Our street, this Einsiedlergasse, bordering on the Hundsturm, used to be the limit, the borderline. On this land I went out and chased about with the *Strizibuben* (kids from the gutter) as they were known. They were not thieves, no, but guttersnipes, real guttersnipes. And when I came home I was punished, yes, I was beaten.

So I climbed down the fire-escape to the street to escape the beating. I can still remember that. I wanted now to go and live among the *Strizibuben*. They were rough and I too was rough and no more would I live that lonely and respectable life in which I was beaten.

Sometimes with my Papa I went from the Einsiedlergasse, where we lived, up into the Arbeitergasse in the evening to the pub. He was always of the opinion that I should be prepared for life, to mingle, because there was still this large differentiation, between our bourgeoisie and the working classes. And so Papa took me with him to the pub, which to Mama's sorrow had evil repercussions, because that's how I learnt the rough and vulgar Viennese dialect. Through that and through the running around with the gutterboys, I learnt the most fearful dialect, so that then my Mama was ashamed of me, and when the relatives came, or when there were visitors she couldn't have me there, because I enjoyed to speak only this dialect. It was a rebellion like in the young today. I did not love the middle class. Already I had a feeling for languages, and I spoke this dialect in such a way that they had to separate me from the visitors. And when I had committed some villainy, and the parents were cross, I fled under the bed in my room and lay in the corner in such a way, so deeply in it and behind it, and kicked so hard with my legs and with my shoes, that they couldn't get me out. Well, they should have hit hard with a whip or God knows what.

But the bed could not be moved. That was good. That was very good. For there I am under it. With my gutter speech. That was one of my salvations, the other was the fire-escape. On the house there was a ladder, so I always fled when I wanted to get away and the doors were closed. I went on to the balcony where they beat carpets, and down the fire-ladder. At the end was a jump, a big jump. This did not worry me. I could hang by my hands and just drop like a plum. When you drop you just relax, then all is well.

Do I give you some idea of how bad a girl I was? Perhaps not bad, but naughty, certainly. It cannot be right always to run away from the home. But my spirit was too proud—or should I say arrogant?—for the insult of beatings, and too shocked, too humiliated, when all I sought was a little diversion that did no harm. At any rate, not much harm. So always I was running away. They had to send the maids and assistants out searching for me and even the police. I was not a delightful child.

A Holy Bitch

In other ways I was bad also. But things went better when I got to the convent school. First I went to the Ursulines in the Johannesgasse; the coachman drove me every morning to the Johannesgasse and there I was tamed a little.

So pious I became! I went to confession, and I was forbidden to run about with the boys who were my friends, the *Strizibuben*. But because of all this piety, to suffer began to seem a holy thing. It was a theatrical experience. Yes, I was a holy bitch, for with my inquisitive nature sometimes I peeped behind the scenes.

And so it was once when we drove to the Tivoli, my parents and I, I carried my prayer-book with me, and in it I had marked all the sins I had committed, as the next morning I was going to the priest for confession, poor him! And my father he looked at the book and read this list of sins and I was beaten really hard in the carriage, as there were practically no sins that I hadn't marked. I was then about eight or nine years old. Yes, I had lied, cheated, stolen.

Yes, I stole. From the shop where the cherries were. At confession the priest told me I must return the cherries. This, naturally I could not do, for I had eaten them all. Then I must return cherries to replace those I had stolen; it was not a lot. So I found more cherries, these I did not steal, and I turned up with the cherries and this fruitseller in the meantime had put a net over the cherries; so few had I been able to steal, yet he knew.

So I chucked the cherries on to the net and I ran away.

Yes, yes, that was naughty. And so you see I had to confess that too. And penance, this too I had to do and had not to laugh, because I could not help thinking the beads of my rosary were cherries and how good it would be to steal some more and not be all the time so holy. And so I became again rebellious, which led to depression, and it is only in depression that you ask God to forgive you, and also request favours.

But the place where I was beaten in the Tivoli because of all the written-down sins, oh! it was lovely there then. It had not been built over as it now is, but there was this large space with trees and a large meadow where you could romp about as a child.

When I went to the Ursulines I never wanted the carriage to wait outside the Convent, as I was dead ashamed in front of the other girls who all came on foot, if I had to get into this beautiful carriage. So the coachman had to stop in the Annagasse and the Convent is by the Johannesgasse.

And then other times we drove down into the Prater

every day at noon. To the *Jause* as it was called, which you call elevenses, no? In the Lusthaus down in the Prater every day at noon. And the meadows in those days were still full of stags and red deer. That was lovely.

I, of course, never stayed in the carriage. Out I got, and ran on foot and never wanted to stay like a good girl with them in the carriage. I went quietly near the red deer, and they looked at me and some of them continued to eat and some moved away. If I sat down and remained still, they returned. I named them all and forgot the names and so did they.

Except Elizabeth, who loved me from a little distance and answered her name by raising her head from grazing to smile at me. But then I discovered her name should have been Franz Josef; my eyes had not looked in those parts to see how it was back there. After this I looked and gave new names. And this reminds me how many times, a little later, I spoilt my quick affairs with boys by laughing. I could not help it. When this thing stuck up. Always I laughed. Like Hell! And then angry they got, and down it went again and all was finished. This I could not help. It is only when I do not look, it goes well and all is fine. *Ja, ja*, so fine it is then.

I told you 'quick affairs' because that is what I have always liked. Quick and finish. Yes; this you may print, it is part of my character.

Now I will tell you a bit more about the school at the Ursulines. There I was until the age of fourteen. Quite a naughty girl and often found out. They only permitted me to stay there because Mama took all those Catholic journals and tracts. Pious I was still, certainly, but naughty, too. No longer did I write down all my sins in order to be beaten at home, I had learnt a little *furberia* (cunning). Never enough. And it is always in this way, I am *furba* only when it does not help and never on the important occasions. So it is with me. So I am.

A Beating in Anacapri

Before I forget everything, I must tell you how I was beaten again many, many years after. As a qualified doctor practising on Capri I was beaten. You laugh, you think I mean just a pam pam on my fat bottom, but this was quite a business. I was beaten by these people at Anacapri, which you know is up on the cliff high above the town of Capri. They came at me and they attacked me with sticks.

It was in this way. In those days I did not have an office, no . . . I went out only on visits, and I had rows, big rows, with my colleagues, because there were two doctors, a Doctor Frogillo in Anacapri and a Doctor Gennaro in Capri, and they discovered that there had come a foreign woman who grabbed many patients away from them, and they became refractory. So I was summoned by the Municipio of Capri and went to the Parish Council and showed them my diploma, and that was the only mistake I had committed—I should have registered with the *Ordine dei Medici* (Medical Council) in Naples. This was done after I had sent in my diploma, and then they issued me with one for Capri, so now I became a resident and then everything was in order. But then this other bad thing happened with the locals, they threatened to kill me.

It was like this. A farmer in Anacapri had a daughter who was dying, a very bad consumptive in the last stage

26

of it, she was not my patient, but everyone called me in (they all did so, 'Come!' they commanded because the other doctors would not come if it was late or they were at dinner or with a woman). When I went there, I just said—I was honest—there was nothing I could do to help, the doctor concerned had perhaps not paid so much attention to so hopeless a case . . . the relatives then became very angry, since, when a young girl had this disease, it was a disgrace for the family in the sense that the other daughters then had difficulties in being married.

Then the colleagues added fuel to the flames . . . the one from Anacapri, he especially. So that he could escape their anger. And then they were against me, as peasants are in such a situation. When one night I returned from a very sick child—it had scarlet fever—from the piazza in Anacapri, I walked across the Piazza Boffe, and I saw these muffled-up figures, the hats jammed low on their heads, it was round about midnight and they called to each other: 'Let's go, let's give it to her.' They had cudgels in their hands and I ran and just made it to my door in time and there I was hit as I inserted the key. Oh, yes, I had blood in my hair.

And in those days I could *really* run; like a monkey, I could even jump on precipices . . . No longer is this possible, only perhaps if I am pursued, for I am strong for an old one. It is the eyes, you see, which cannot discern enough with the climbing and how you must find the ledges and (do you say?) grip-holds. So I ran, and they ran. And they lost all their breath chasing me and calling: 'Now we get her!' and I lost mine not at all, and so I arrived at my door just in time while they started to hit. Yes, a good boum-pouff on the head, yes, blood there was and pouff-boum on my shoulders. Then I kicked at them, at their knees and other places which you should not kick, and I kicked my way in and slammed the door and locked the key and the chain and the bolts and all what there was. Yes, with bolts and a bar and a chain. And I was wild, I was so angry, I would have run out again and lashed at them, but I had not a lash. I was frightened, really frightened, but worse was the disgust. The disgust is when they come together more than one, when no longer do they think as one, when they have decided together on destroying one who is alone and cannot defend her life. It is when they are no longer thinking as individuals but turning into savages all together.

In a religious procession this is another affair! There are in religious processions faces that are made beautiful, and hypocritical faces, those are a joke, and faces that are just quiet. There is in a religious procession more love than hate, and the purpose is love, not hate, and some *really* worship. But hate—hate disgusts me. A bad illness it is. To be angry, to be really furious, sometimes that is necessary. Then all is over. You may be rid of it; pouf! Hate is quite another thing.

The Archduke

Now I will tell you about Vienna and the ice and the winters. The Danube is *never* blue, so yellow it is, all frozen. I climbed on to it and people of course fetched me off it, but I had a slide first. How fine, *Santa Madonna*! Fast like Hell! And so, of course, I was again beaten. But otherwise it was lovely.

Those were real winters. One could always skate on

the old Danube. The temperatures were around minus 14 to minus 16 degrees of frost. The whole winter long. Also the small lakes in the Prater were always frozen.

Mama drove with Uncle. Because he no longer practised and he was an old gentleman and they drove together, in the winter with the sledge and in the summer in the carriage. I can also remember, as I told you already, there were lots of invalids, so many galloping consumptives. When one drove through the streets, there were a lot of houses in front of which lay straw piled up, to dampen the noise. Everything, the pavement, as well as the street, was covered in straw. When there was snow and sledges, no, but at other times.

In the spring, it was beautiful with violets in the Prater. That really was lovely. Real violets. Not what you are thinking, the prostitutes; they too were there. Yes, many; a waiting-list.

And then May came and there was the Battle of Flowers in the Prater. One carriage after another and all the carriages garlanded. Everyone drove in it, in landaulettes. In the big carriages, the horses were decked in flowers and the whips and the coachmen, and behind the horses the decorated carriages, wonderful; they drove down one side of the Prater to the Lusthaus, and up the other side back again. And the sidewalks were crammed with spectators.

Archduke Salvator drove and the others, the relevant ladies, drove in the carriages with the relevant liveries. One or two or three from the Royal Court drove in the procession. It was like an honorary free gift to us all, that they too drove with the rest. And I stood with Mama where the trees are. There was no trellis and nothing fenced in. You know what the Prater is like in the Hauptallee, and I was given such lovely flowers. A lady had given Mama the flowers, and I took the flowers away from Mama, and I can remember exactly as I stood there (you could see down to the Tegetthoff Monument) they said: 'Now, NOW here he is! The Archduke!' And as he came nearer and nearer I ran forward, through the horses, right up to the carriage and threw the flowers. I don't know whether into his lap or hers. So quickly I did this thing (imagine if there had been a bomb in them!) and I only know that he laughed a great deal. Mama blushed hard and pleaded with her hands as though begging forgiveness. There was no police, there was no one as guard, it wasn't like that in those days. The people cried, 'Look at that child, that child,' and then it was all over. That I can still remember.

With the Nuns

At the Convent I did primary school and secondary school, till I was nearly fourteen. I was also a naughty child at the Ursulines, quite a bad girl, yes, yes, and was often found out. Once I threw an old gentleman down because when school was over I pushed too hard to get out; those who were walking in front of me fell on to the old gentleman and he fell too and how sorry I was; no more could he move. He said, 'My children you are so full of life you don't need mine.' And so he laughed and the girls they helped him up. He had not broken anything. He had just sat down on his popo. Then in the break in the Convent I threw snowballs at the sisters. This is true, yes. My parents didn't have an easy time of it.

As soon as I was through secondary school, they put me into Notre Dame des Nations Convent, near the Ulrichskirche. They put me in there and everything was very French. I had to learn the ancient history of the Middle Ages in French, and I did this entirely by ear. And by ear I could recite my lessons. I could recite that which I had read, but I didn't understand anything. And that's why my memory was so well trained that in later years, a biography of Schiller which had two and a half pages, I had to read it once, and then I could get up and spout it from beginning to end.

Of course the nuns discovered this. Nuns always discover. My parents had already told them that I couldn't speak a word of French and they didn't speak German.

Half the Balkans sent their daughters there. Rumanians, Serbs, Bulgarians, they sent their children away from home to Notre Dame. And I became so Catholic that I was forever confessing and wanted an altar at home, and what was worse, I wanted to become a nun.

I was fifteen when I wanted to become a nun, and when Papa forbade me this, I went on a ten-day hunger strike. I ate nothing. Until the doctor came and said that Papa had to go to the country with me immediately. It was only May, but nevertheless into the country we went. They drove me to St Wolfgang. The doctor said, 'When she gets away from this convent, then she will give up the idea,' therefore, a change of climate there must be, because they couldn't get me to break my hunger strike. I was too passionate, I insisted on becoming a nun and I thought I could get my way by striking and Papa would give in.

Well . . . it went wrong. Now you'll laugh . . . I had hardly been in St Wolfgang a few weeks, and there was no more talk of nuns. I ran away from home and went around with the Pater boys, they were the sons of the Hotel Pater, there were four boys and a girl, Henriette, and the four boys had a boat and I learnt to swim and nearly got drowned the first time, and then with the sailing I got under the boat when we capsized. And when autumn came and we returned home there was of course no more talk of becoming a nun. Not a word.

It was a lovely summer, but for my parents it was not so good because they were always afraid because of the lake, that I would drown. We capsized right in front of the steamer, so there was a lot of fuss and the lifeboat had to come and save us. Another time we went up a mountain and stayed the night without saying where we were going and the next day they sent people up to see . . . With being a nun it was all finished, and my vocation, do you call it, was quite gone away.

In the autumn they said I should stay home nice and good and help Mama with the housekeeping, dusting . . . but that was not for me. I said, I want to learn something. So I got a state diploma which allowed me to give lessons. I learnt all this in the language school Weiser.

First I led a small children's course. I taught French and English. And with the money which I earned with French and English lessons, and my pocket money on top of that, I enrolled for a two-year preparation with Schwarzwald's for the school-leaving certificate. I did it all myself, and had to chase about Vienna. Then my parents gave in when they realised I was ruining my health with giving lessons.

There was never any talk about going into the hairdressing business, because that was no longer ours.

Mama stayed with the uncles in Einsiedlergasse. She went no more to dress hair, but looked after the old gentlemen. Papa, for a while, went on with the shop, but then he broke his collar-bone and because of that he had to give up and live on his earnings. He busied himself with the sale and buying of houses and such things. No longer with his profession. His two brothers who came from Germany took over the shop. He had two younger brothers and he handed over both shops. The one in the Singerstrasse, and a new one in the Weihburggasse. The one in the Weihburggasse is still as it was. Many years ago, my uncle, his name was Hermann Klaeser, ran this. And the other uncle, André, was first in the Singerstrasse and then went to the Hotel Bristol, a very grand hotel. He was then hairdresser in the Hotel Bristol, and his daughters are still alive, one is an actress and lives out in Huetteldorf.

First Love

So there I was in the Schwarzwald school, and at first I was naughty again. I met a young girl, a certain Frieda Abeles, a Jewess, whom I really got fond of, and she lived with her relatives, Adler by name, in the Leopoldstadt, and with the son, Max Adler . . .

Yes, how shall I explain this to you? It was not a question of courting—in those days we didn't court. Courting! What a waste of time! We went about together when we were free, without my parents' knowledge. When the Schwarzwald class ended, we went up on the Albrechtsrampe, and had our fun up there. And when Mama arrived later and waited for me at the school down below, we could see her come and even spit on her. She had no idea we were up there, and the spit didn't go so far down, and she looked all over the place for me. It was first love, yes. (Before that as a child, I only had my cousin with whom I ran around a little in Lainz, but that was a childish story, even though the sin register I carried in the carriage was so full.)

Max Adler was my age, between nineteen and twenty. I had been to language school, and after language school, I was teaching grown-up people. In one way, of course, we were both of us completely grown-up. So that first love went on on the Albrechtsrampe and when it was dark, in the Schillerpark. The Schillerpark is in front of the Akademie, and we sat on benches in the twilight. That was first love, yes, big sins many times, so fine it was. My parents didn't know that, but they apprehended it. Perhaps not all of it. Not how bad it was and how good. First, they only thought I was with my friend Frieda Abeles, but then they discovered, well . . . that there was someone also.

We went to the opera. I can remember there was quite a to-do at the opera. We went with Max. And Caruso was there. And at the second or third performance I couldn't get a ticket, they were all sold out, but I determined to see Caruso without fail, and I squeezed through at the ticket control without a ticket, and of course, after the first act, they grabbed me and took me down to the inspector, Madl by name, to the chief inspector . . . and they said, well, to be sure, as I queued every day for the opera, and because I went every day . . . that was an extenuating circumstance, and then Madl said, 'All the same this is a very bad story.' And so at home I got a summons and I went to the police station, but the police inspector there said, 'I don't want to spoil your whole career for you. You are a student in the Gymnasium and are about to take your Matura (leaving certificate) and shall I spoil it all for you with this summons?' It was well with him and he was kind to me.

You see I wanted above everything in the world to hear Caruso sing. It was wonderful. You have no conception. He sang in the Verdi operas, *Trovatore*, and *Traviata*, and then I heard him in all the tenor roles. He was small and fat and very lively and he sang . . . how he sang. From the time I got my Matura till I had my doctorate I went every night to the opera. Every night. Either to the opera or to the Burgtheater.

A Sort of Hotel

It was then I had this thing about Josef Kainz. We stood at the stage door and brought him carnations. Yes . . . that was a real crush. His acting was like no one else's.

Once we were at the stage door and waited for Kainz who played in *The Jewess from Toledo*, but it was Hoffmann who came out first. Hoffmann was a young actor whom I had met, and he said: 'Now we will go and eat, let's go to the Tiefer Graben, there is a nice hotel, and there we can kiss and be together.' So I went with him. And that was the first time I realised that that sort of hotel existed, and that one can go to them, like that, not to sleep, no!

At the porter's I was very ashamed. Because he must have noticed I was very young, and then probably he knew Hoffmann already, because he probably had brought others he had known in the theatre. Afterwards Max Adler was very cross with me. But afterwards we also went, because Hoffmann had given us the idea, not to the same hotel, to another one of the same sort somewhere in the Ringstrasse. And we had dates that on this or that day we would go again. So that it got to be quite a habit, this hotel-going, and all would not have happened if that man Hoffmann hadn't come out of the theatre door before Kainz. So it always is. So it was later in Positano. You expect one man, and then pouf! it is another. But to tell you the truth it wasn't the same feeling which I had then as I had later. It was a hurlyburly, it was no deep pleasure. It was a kind of rehearsal, a game. But I certainly felt important that I went now to hotels . . .

I was still very young. Perhaps in that time all girls were a lot better behaved than I was. I don't really know, but in middle-class circles the daughters were very shielded. It was only I who was such a specimen, not like now when they all do it. We were formed through religion as also by the milieu in which we grew up, and we never had the opportunity. They didn't let a young girl go about alone with anyone. Not two paces did they go. But those who wanted to very much like me could achieve it. One had to have a very strong determination.

Today I read, to the accompaniment of a February storm, the letters which my parents wrote to one another during their period of engagement. How hard life must have been then. Such serious letters. How dreadful, that only now, so many years after their death, I am beginning to understand them. Why did they never have contact with their only child, as I have contact with my children? It was, I suppose, still the other generation, there was only a little love, and less trust.

Today I also read the letter from Vienna, from the poor-relief hospital, with a rebuke that I, her only child, was letting my mother die in the hospital. How it came to that is no longer clear to me. I had brought her to Capri, to me, with all her furniture, but she suffered from the surroundings, because of course she could not talk to anyone except me, even my children spoke Italian. She couldn't understand the sermon in church, nor go to confession, and she was so very religious, and the heat in the summer she couldn't stand at all. She wanted to go back to Vienna, and I agreed, which I should never have done, because I should have thought that she would be alone there and die there, which last was her wish after all, because she wanted to be laid in the tomb with husband and relatives, there to rest. But only now when I am old, and so very alone and live in my house with my dog, only now can I grasp how much my poor mother must have suffered and it hurts me in my heart and I am unconsolable about it, and keep thinking why I never really loved my mother. In my youth she was always a drag on all my strivings, she didn't want me to study, and she opposed my marriage.

The Big Time

It was a big time, yes, in Vienna with the theatre and the opera. There were Schmedes and Slezak, and then there was Winkelmann. At his farewell, we took the horses out of his carriage and pulled him all along the Ring. I can remember Mama sent the maid to fetch me because at that time we already lived far out, and she was afraid for me to be alone. There were a lot of petty thieves there who pinched one's earrings or one's popo.

Then of course I saw Duse. She was fine, fine, yes. Really great and (how shall I say?) she went straight to the heart. A really big contrast with other actresses. I often went to the Burgtheater and saw Hohenfels, everyone knew Hohenfels, but Duse, that was something quite different . . . not only because she was Italian; the gestures, the enunciation, the whole thing was a sensation.

It was no longer with Max Adler that I went. There was no Max Adler any more. He was only for a while, that boy, at the beginning. I think he went to work in the Allgemeine Bankverein and became a bank clerk. He is alive or he has died. I do not know. I only know he showed up once when I was on holiday in Grossgmain. He was there when I won the tennis tournament. For the ladies singles, a prize. A lovely turned-silver, what does one call it, oh yes, manicure set. He came specially to see me play. But then it was already over between us.

Studying Medicine

My Matura examination I took in Salzburg, at the Gymnasium, not in Vienna. My maths were so weak, I couldn't be taught, even with memory, in maths. I just couldn't. I took a crammer—but it didn't work. But in Salzburg I got distinction in all subjects and in maths, 'Good'. They asked me what I wanted to study, and I said I wanted to study medicine. This had impressed me already as a child, and they let me through by a majority vote but not unanimously.

38

When I was through with the Matura, we were once in the Volksgarten, and there came one of the students, a medical student whose name was Klaar. I said, 'I doubt if I will make a doctor because it is so disgusting because of the corpses.' So he took me with him from the Volksgarten on a lovely afternoon at five o'clock to the Institute of Anatomy and took me down where the corpses lie in cauldrons, and I did not turn a hair. I was quite resistant, that part was OK. So now I thought I can peacefully study medicine, and I registered for the medical course.

There were only two girls among the students, and I was one. It was a nightmare for my parents—all these studies at the Schwarzwald school, this going to the opera, Max Adler, the Matura—my whole life was a nightmare to them. When, on top of that, they heard I was going to study medicine, Uncle was called, and as a big girl I was beaten really hard. And, as you have seen, punishment only made my will like iron.

He was a very determined man, this uncle, and with my probably rude answers and my not good behaviour, he must have got angry too, and he was a very strong man, but I was after all, well, yes, twenty. 'I'll drive that out of you, this is indecent in our family . . .' Papa joined him and they both yelled, 'In our family we don't want such a one, who is *impazzata* with the boys, it is only so that you can sit around with the boys.'

That's how they looked on it then. For a girl to study medicine was to be despised. We were the only two girls. Me and the Jewess, Frieda. There was no one else.

I studied with Tandler. I was very popular with Tandler. He wanted me later to become a demonstrator in the Anatomy Department, and he always took my part. Everything was always fine with the studies, only maths, but I didn't need maths any more.

You think I am tired? I am not tired when I talk; I plod on like a camel.

Another Affair

Now we come to another affair. My parents who wanted no part of these studies, took me to balls. There were so many of them, and at one I became friendly with a certain Lieutenant Rehn. A good-looking boy. He was invited to the house, there were teas to which a lot of people were invited, and there was this Lieutenant Rehn, and then I was supposed to marry this Lieutenant. And my Papa said there was security because he had a job, and my father told Mama, let her get married, but it was not good, because I was obstinate, I didn't want to. I had no feelings for him. The idea of giving up my studies to marry this Rehn—oh, for heaven's sake, no, I was revolted. So when he was invited, I always went out before he came. You see how I was, how I always have been. When I do not want something, it is no go. Nothing to be done. So I am, so I will always be. Mama noticed finally that it was no good. So then of course there were eternal rows. 'You only want to run around with this Max Adler and this is indecent.'

But now I was at university, there was no more that boy Adler, it went differently now. At the Matura in Salzburg I had met a certain Norbert Baudisch.

Norbert Baudisch was the son of a civil servant in Salzburg. He had a good position. This Norbert Baudisch fell in love with me, and I fell in love with him. My parents had rented a house for the summer in Grossgmain near Salzburg and Baudisch always came to visit me . . . so I had this little love affair with Baudisch, which my parents more or less countenanced. 'Well,' they thought, 'he is studying medicine also, he is not that Adler, so that is a little better. She thinks this is the one now and they may surely, later, get married.' Perhaps that is what they believed, although I never thought of marrying, nor did he. I did not have these domestic ideas, mine were quite independent, but this affair at least was something which the parents thought they understood. A lot of nonsense because they could understand it as little as everything that had happened before.

Tandler always teased me about Baudisch, and I was very naughty in the dissecting room once, because with the syringe with which one syringes the corpses I sprayed everyone, and the professor only just got out of the door in time. It was all because of that man, Baudisch. I tell you, the Dottoressa has always been an impossible woman.

Then I went on holiday. My parents in this instance had a lot of confidence in me, which was quite unfounded, and I don't know why they had this confidence, because I went with Baudisch to Florence.

It came about like this. We went into the Alps down into Doblach, or whatever this is called, into South Tyrol. It was a mountaineering party. That parents accept. But when the mountaineering party was over we sat ourselves down in a train, the two of us, as we wanted to see Italy and go to Florence.

In Florence I went to the Pensione Daddi. My parents told me to go there, but Norbert Baudisch was also in the pensione and that they did not know. And we went to the Giardini Boboli and whatever else one does in Florence, and afterwards we came back like good children.

Of course I rushed into all the museums. I only spoke a little Italian then. Not too much, only that Italian which one knows from grammar books. Anyway it was more than Baudisch. He didn't know a word. Yes, it was the first time in Italy and Italy didn't make such a big impression on me. The next year in the vacation, I travelled further, I went to Rome, but I was not with Baudisch. No, no . . . that was already different.

It was with one called Tolleg I was in Rome next year. He was a Frenchman. A tiny little man. Still quite young. A painter. Well, not really a painter. A caricaturist. He was a sickly person. A poor devil he was. That I remember. And with him I went to the Café Greco and to all those things and to the museums. Then there was another colleague, Doctor Beck, whom I still see. He was in Rome too and he was very interested in Tolleg, and they became great friends.

I, on the other hand, could not stand this Rome or this Tolleg and I went all alone to Palermo. It fascinated me so. In Naples I was for a short time, and went on to Palermo, and that was my first encounter with Sicily, which impressed me greatly. I travelled from Palermo directly back to Vienna to my studies, and I no longer wanted Tolleg. Things had changed. Beck looked after Tolleg and brought Tolleg back to Vienna and then sent Tolleg comfortably to Paris, where he found something good and where he landed in the right circles. I never heard anything further from him. The studies progressed and I had a lot of colleagues whom I liked—

Schallinger, Hirschenhauser, and Italian Leonardo who came from Bolzano, Baudisch of course also, and then later Doctor Mund, a Pole, whom I loved greatly then. He was killed in the first world war.

A Certain Alfons

The study of medicine can be very depressing because of the many difficult cases of internal medicine. So I moved for a semester into zoology and listened to lectures given by Professor Werner, that is I went on with the practicals at the Institute of Anatomy, only without doing the internal studies. Whenever possible I did zoology with Professor Werner. In the afternoons I went on excursions into the Vienna woods. How beautiful it was, and in this year there was the comet. What comet I don't remember—it doesn't matter. It was good to look at it from the Hapsburgwarte, in the evening, lovely to see. The tail was so brilliant. It was full moon and people were afraid. The simple people in the street said the world was going to end. Such fear there was. After a couple of days they got used to it. Like pigeons alarmed by a gun. Soon they are strutting after their food again.

At that time I had a new colleague who also studied zoology, a certain Alfons Gabriel, the son of an officer. He lived in the Hasenauerstrasse out in Doebling and he had such enthusiasm for his zoology that he fired me with it. He liked to go to Wagner operas, and so there we were once again in the Vienna woods and in the evening we went to the *Valkyrie*, but we brought with us from the woods a frog in a bottle. It was May or June; a frog in a bottle and just in the *piano* of the duet between Siegmund and Sieglinde, that frog had to start croaking. The people surrounding us in the gallery looked, and Alfi said like the others, 'Be quiet, shush,' so no one could know what place the animal was croaking from. You see we had these specimen bottles into which one puts the animals one finds. He was probably very uncomfortable in the bottle, so he started croaking. It probably had never happened before that a frog started croaking in the midst of that elegant *pianissimo* singing. It could only happen to us.

Alfons and I decided, if it were at all possible, to make an African journey. Well, he stayed the course and later became an African explorer. We wanted to go to Tunis in the summer. It was the closest bit of Africa which we could see. So Tunis it was, let's go to Tunis. Professor Werner from the Department of Zoology said, 'If in the summer you get to Tunis you must bring me such and such a butterfly.' He had a collection of butterflies and he didn't have some of the ones which apparently one could catch only in Tunisia, and so he said, 'You can't go to Tunis just for the fun of it. If you're going there, if it is at all possible, you will catch me these butterflies.'

Well, we went, and we took this equipment just in case, so that we could bring the stuff as far as Vienna to prepare them. There was at that time a direct train, it doesn't exist any more, from Vienna via Salerno to Sicily. Now you must change all the time, unless you take some express *di gran' lusso* which is too *aristocratisch* for me. And so we went from Vienna as far as Salerno, and got out in Salerno, because at Positano there was my school friend about whom I have told you, Frieda Abeles. But what I forgot to tell you was

44

how once in the Gymnasium, in a fury, I dragged her by her long plaits right through the classroom. They threatened to expel me, because this was gross cruelty you see. But she, she was such an impudent one, and she gave me such cheeky answers to everything I said to her. Cutting, cheeky answers which annoyed me, so I grabbed her two plaits and there was such a yelling, and the other girls screamed also, and the professor came, and I was dragged to the Head. And then they said if that happened again, out they would push me. And I had to apologise, and I did it, though why should I apologise? for after all she was my friend, but she was always so insufferable.

All the same I liked her far too much. I was jealous of her sometimes, when she spent much more time with others than with me. There was perhaps a certain rivalry in me, because I reacted like that, I think. This good Frieda Abeles had been in Florence, and in Florence had met a certain Doctor Ritzenfeld who was studying archaeology, and a certain Gigi Moor, an artist.

Meeting Gigi Moor

Gigi was the son of the director of State railways in Basel and he was a painter. In painting he was still very young. He was only eighteen. He had run away from his parents, and he joined up with this Alfred Ritzenfeld because he came from his home-town, and I don't suppose the family supported him, and so he gave violin lessons in Florence. And they were both friends of my girl friend, Frieda Abeles, and they got together and they all three went from Florence down to Positano. Today Positano is *too* well known, like Capri or the

Riviera, but then it was just a fishing village. In Positano they had rented a house, with a beautiful terrace, with a piano where they gave concerts. Ritzenfeld could play the piano well, and Gigi, he played the violin.

Gigi was a good-looking lad. In Positano he was known as *Gigi 'o bello*. A very beautiful eighteen-year-old boy; there they were, and Frieda, she had written to me in Vienna: 'If you really want to go to Tunis, why don't you stop by, we have this house here, so do come and visit us.' Well, I got out of the train at Salerno with my friend. With this Alfons Gabriel. And we arrived in Positano with the steamer.

You cannot land in Positano; you have to get a rowing-boat to go alongside the steamer, and in this rowing-boat there was of course Gigi. Tall, sunburnt, wearing only a bathing slip, he helped the passengers who were arriving into the boat, and then he introduced himself and said he had come from Frieda Abeles. 'You just come with me now, we are waiting for you.' And then I presented my friend Alfons Gabriel, 'So you both come with us,' and then he introduced Ritzenfeld and he said, 'We won't stay on this beach, we'll go to the other beach, the Pornillo beach, it's much more pleasant there.' That was the time in Positano when the young bathed naked. The young men that is. Not the women. On the contrary the women wore a lot of clothes, but the men, and above all the young men, the youths, bathed naked, and so the Pornillo beach was a lot more cosy. And then they took me to their house. We got there from the Marina Grande, a lovely house with a large terrace. So I said to Alfi, 'This is going to be lovely here, yes, we'll fix everything.'

All at once the good Gigi disappeared and Ritzen-

46

feld said, 'He's going to the Chiesa Nuova, that's above us, and he is going to fetch his fiddle down, and then we will play you something lovely, and I will bring a skipping-rope with me and we can skip on the terrace.' So we skipped. And I can remember exactly how it grew darker, and then the piano concerto followed which they played to me, I think it was Bach, I don't remember exactly; anyway they played me a concerto with lovely candles on the piano, because there was no electric light.

Evening came. And they said, let's get on with the skipping. 'It's no good,' Alfi said, 'it is already dark on the terrace,' and then he said he was tired, for tomorrow we wanted to go to Capri. 'I want to see Capri if I'm here.' So he went away from us and he went to sleep. But I remained with the good Gigi and that was the first night of loving him. It was love at first sight. A real love at first sight. The first *big* love.

He was very dark and tall. Everyone said he was far above others in beauty, better than Rudolph Valentino and all those actors they raved about. Very young, eighteen years old, and I was already twenty-four. It was all very lovely. When you are young, you expect many wonders, but I can tell you now, when I am such an old one, how very rare they are.

So it was that in the morning I said to Alfi: 'Well, well, you go to Capri and look at Capri. I am going to stay here for two days.'

Frieda Abeles did not say anything. She had the other—Ritzenfeld. She liked Gigi, but he could not stand her. No!

Only the other day my friend Doctor Beck said: 'I'll tell you something.' At the time when Alfred Ritzenfeld and Gigi were in Florence, they were in quite some money trouble and Alfred said, 'I shall go to Rome and see if I can't pick up something,' and then he went to Rome and at the *Piccolo Uomo*, that was a restaurant, he met Frieda Abeles, and after a short time, there came a telegram for Gigi, to Florence, 'Jewess found, come.' So it was she lived with both of them, do you understand, in the villa in Positano. I should be grateful to her. Well, yes, that is the truth. She found for me first Max Adler and then Gigi.

So I was there, but I could only stay two days as I had to go away, and travel with Alfi. But Gigi at the moment he didn't understand that I had with Alfi a purely friendly relationship. That is true, what I say, yes.

It was like that from the beginning. Zoological studies and excursions in the Vienna woods, and then together to the Oriental Institute in the afternoons to prepare ourselves in Arabic because we thought when we got to Tunis, we should at least be able to speak a few words of Arabic. So you see, this was an entirely scientific and platonic relationship. And probably Alfi never grasped that I had fallen in love at first sight with this Gigi; that it had become a *real* love affair. That he didn't know.

We went to Tunis. In Tunis it was quite pleasant for a few days, but already we said, 'No! In Tunis alone there is nothing, we won't stay here,' and so we went by train to Tabarka. Tabarka is a place on the Mediterranean on the coast of Tunis towards Algiers.

We went there by train and there was a very lonely place opposite, a tiny island. A very tiny island. And there we went with the butterfly-net to the beach (it wasn't a bathing beach but a wild beach), there to catch these butterflies, and over to the small island to which one could almost swim, so close it was. But the fishermen took us in a boat fast over to the island and there were mice that came (so rarely was it visited): lovely mice, yes, they came to us quite tame and let us feed them, they knew no people. It was very lovely there on this beach.

However, now there was a fight with Alfi. It came to a quarrel, because he wanted to go further, to the Bay of Gabes on the instruction of Professor Werner, so that one should seek there those butterflies. And sand-beetles. We were to collect them, and that was too much for me, it went against the grain because I wanted to go to Cairo (too far) and to Gafsa and Tozeur. Near Cairo there are beautiful temples, and there were the oases and I wanted to see them, Nefta too, and he was only interested in this Gabes, and I said, 'No, no, now that I am in Tunis I want to see all this, not damned butterflies!' He refused, so I sent a telegram to Baudisch, my friend, who was spending the vacation in the South of France, and he took a ship in Marseilles and travelled to Tunis and picked me up and I went with him to Gafsa first and then Tozeur and Nefta which has naked boys who dive from the trees which grow over the pools. Damned butterflies! Leave the poor beasts to enjoy their short life.

Alfi was of course very offended. But Baudisch was happy, because to him this journey with Alfi had been a thorn in his eye. I use the right expression?

Anyway I left Alfi. Now excuse me, I use your bathroom.

But all this time the beautiful Gigi stayed in Positano. We hadn't made any definite arrangements. He knew I was a student, and that after this trip I would return to Vienna, because that was only a summer vacation.

I was in the Oasis of Gafsa, which I liked a lot. Above all in the evening with the Arabs at the tables where they drank their coffee, and smoked their pipes, and then from there we went somewhere far lovelier: Nefta, which is an oasis with beautiful date palms and pomegranates and a cold spring. I had not imagined it like that. An oasis with a lovely cold spring, which one could jump into and swim. It was delicious when we arrived in the evening straight from the terribly overheated train . . .

One left Tunis at midday and one was there towards evening. On the way, the Bedouins got on after they had said their prayers, and as night began to fall the train halted, and all the people got down and lay down on their carpets and said their prayers, then they got in again and the train went on. It was funny how their noses went down on the sand and their bottoms up in the air.

They seemed to pay little attention to us foreigners, they did not bother us. Only in Tabarka there had been a young boy round twelve years old, who made friends with me and wanted to know how it was over in Europe: he always spoke about Marseilles, would I not take him with me when I went away? And would I not go into the bushes with him?

He wanted to seduce me, that twelve-year-old brat, so I bonked him one. You know they are completely shaven, except for one curl, and the young ones have the curl tied up with a ribbon, a blue ribbon. And I bonked him because into the bushes he wanted I should go. You can imagine how Baudisch laughed. 'Such cheek!' he said.

What am I saying now? It was not yet Baudisch on the island—it was Alfi. Baudisch, Alfi, Gigi—so many men. So much confusion. And this boy. You say I told you once I did go into the bushes with him. Perhaps you are right. I do not remember. One time perhaps. He was such a little one it could not count, could it? And Alfi he was more outraged by the boy than Baudisch would have been. He was such a dry stick, Alfi. Yes, a scientist; an officer's son, Jesus God, very correct.

The only other thing I can still remember about Gafsa was that in the hotel I had a big scare: on the sheet and on the window-sill there were lots of yellow scorpions running about. I hadn't imagined it like that. And I was even more frightened, when we went out and drank coffee, and they brought a child from the house opposite, a child of about two years, who had been stung by a scorpion, and all this heat too in August. I could not help the child. That was contrary to the law. I yelled out loud: 'Fetch the doctor.' It was I who told them to fetch the doctor. And they fetched the doctor. They told me the next day that the doctor had reported that the child's bottom was too small for such a large scorpion bite. In those days one was not yet used to have these injections against poisonous snakes and such things. One was not so advanced as nowadays.

And then I remember in Nefta the large fountains, they were so lovely. We leapt into them of course, and they were so cool. And then in the evening we were advised we should go out like all the Bedouins; we should travel to one of the warm springs in the desert. So we got into a small carriage, a kind of horsedrawn omnibus, tiny and primitive, with about ten to twelve men in it, all Bedouins, and we drove into the desert around evening, and just as it became dark we arrived at this hot spring. And there were two large swimming basins, two large fountains, one very big, and one quite small, and in the little one there were muffled figures, and that was the women who were bathing, but completely dressed. No, they did not undress, they just went into the water. It was hot. But we, Baudisch and I, we could undress, they gave us a partition. One could go behind a wooden partition and undress and then we could go into the basin with the men, that's what they told Baudisch, if I were not afraid of the men, and in his own fashion he replied: 'You can't scare *her*!' That was after all not true, for when I saw all those dreadful men that night I was scared stiff. Well, I got in all the same, but I suffered agonies of fear that one of them would grab me. After a bit they no longer looked at me like in the bus, friendly. On the contrary they looked at me, not malevolently, but like men look at women. But nothing happened. No one grabbed me. I didn't stay long. The water wasn't hot, it was lukewarm, it was lovely, but I only stayed a few minutes. I had the impression it was debilitating. It must have been some sort of sulphur spring. Because we were deadly tired afterwards.

We returned and got into a bus. This one was open. Like a carriage. There you sat, and the Bedouins, they appeared to be all men, seemed to have got new energy from the bath, and they began to sing. Yes, they sang all their songs, but beautifully, very beautifully. The good Baudisch went to sleep next to me. I suppose he was too exhausted by the bathing . . . But I listened to them . . .

When we got to Gafsa they all of them got out and each one went his way. I made the acquaintance of one of the Bedouins during the next few days. He had a big house with a large plantation, not really large, but for an oasis it was large. He showed me his gardens and his fruit and everything, and tried to persuade me to stay there. He could speak a little French. So I told him better not, for he had also introduced me to his wife. That was nothing to do with it, he said, he would send her away. Yes, yes, I shouldn't worry about her, he would now love me. He would love me and I should stay and he would show me other things and we could go travelling . . . No, no, I said. I got quite scared, such an immense Arab, no! no! That was one of the times I said No. Not often it happened so, like the song we had in Vienna in the old days.

> To the maiden says the Styrian boy,
> What shall I give you now?
> A violet or a carnation plant,
> I will love you, for the rest of my life,
> If you will show me your thighs,
> Right up to where you pee.
> Go stow it, says the maid thereto,
> If I do this, you'll get it for free.

He said we should go on to Tozeur. That is the out-post from where the caravan goes across the Sahara. So Baudisch and I, we went. Tozeur is much more desolate because there are no springs and only small huts.

One went anywhere, and one could eat anywhere, but the food was impossible.

On the return journey I felt so sick, and in these trains there are all those primitive carriages, open, and all of them without any lavatory, nothing, one squatted where the railway carriage ended, one sat down and it just fell down behind you. Terrible, terrible. Anyhow, for the men it didn't matter, but for me it was uncomfortable to hold myself in. The train shook quite a bit, and for me to do it like that! They were very decent, they all went forward in the carriage and no one watched me. But nevertheless it was uncomfortable. First I waited, because I thought I might nip off when the train stopped and do it then. But that was not possible for others got in and some got out again. And then Baudisch told me, 'If you run off now you might be left behind, and we can't communicate. Get on with it and do it like they do, go on, do it like them. Finished.'

We went back to Tunis. We brought back with us two more things from there; a chameleon which I acquired from the woman who sold vegetables in the market in Tunis out of compassion. I felt so sorry for it, and then she said: 'I'll give it to you.' She didn't even sell it to me. She just gave it to me like that. We took it with us. Yes. And we took a hedgehog. It was an African hedgehog. They don't have such short ears like our hedgehogs, but long ears like an elephant. Beautiful long ears. And so I thought, we'll take him with us. We'll show him to Professor Werner.

Alfi *did* bring him some of his butterflies too. Of course Alfi's butterflies were much more valuable than our hedgehog and the chameleon.

Steerage with the Cows

Alfi was still in Gabes—I had no news of him—so Baudisch and I took ship in Tunis for Malta. We were in the steerage class with the cows, because our money was pretty nearly all gone. There was a little sack I had brought from Vienna with gold twenty franc pieces—a whole pouch full, all gold pieces. But they were a little on the wane and so we went steerage to Malta with the cows. But we were very happy and said, 'Thank God we took steerage,' because in the third class there were such dreadful types of Jews and Arabs, and a ghastly rabble which would have been too rough even for me. A dirty, stinking, impossible mob. On the other hand, in the steerage class there were only cows! Well, anyway we sat down on the side where the cows hadn't done their business. And thus we travelled to Malta. Afterwards, all those beautiful, patient eyes stayed with me as if they were still regarding us. And we came to Malta, arriving at Valetta.

It was wonderful in Valetta. The best thing were the fantastic oranges, Malta oranges. Quite small but very sweet, and so good one could eat as many as possible without getting affected by them. It was the pure juice of them, the pure juice. Apart from that the landscape in Malta was beautiful. We had a very fierce storm while we were there.

I forgot to tell you that when we were in the ship, we had a storm on the voyage, and we had a storm in the desert too, on the return journey to Tunis. It was supposed to be a very small one, but nevertheless! The Arabs were all right, they wrapped themselves in their burnouses and were absolutely covered, but all we had was our handkerchiefs and our jackets over the top of us. The sand got into our noses and mouths all the same. If this was only a little storm, it was, you might say, a concentrated essence of a big one. They insisted it was a little storm only, a passing one, a thing of ten minutes, but it was quite bad enough and left behind *such* a rough sea, *Mama mia*!

When we left Malta for Messina we had a very stormy sea again. In the same ship with the same cows. I can still remember how we rolled backwards and forwards. The cows were so restless that I was a little afraid. The sailors pulled us behind a partition on the side where we could huddle together, because they were afraid we might be injured by the cows, that they might get bad-tempered, and thus we arrived in Messina with all the mooing cows which made me laugh.

But Messina, poor destroyed Messina! It was the year after the earthquake. It made a terrifying impression, and so pitiful, though not at first. When we landed our exclamation was: 'The city's still standing.' Yes, but that was all there was, only façades against the sea. All the palaces stood there, and, on arriving, it seemed not so bad, but when you got on land and went behind, everything was empty. Everything. All was gone. There were only walls. Some high, some low. Behind the street, there were only stones. All was down. The city was devastated in such a way, it looked as if giants had jumped on it. There were barracks at one end of Messina and barracks at the other end, and in these were the survivors like ghosts. In other parts the shelters were as primitive as could be. And there were ships. One had to reach the shore first by climbing on to an English ship, and then from this ship one could get on the land. We were there for an afternoon and one night only, and for the night we had to go back to the ship. We couldn't have spent the night on land. How cruel this had been!

We spoke with the people. There we could talk because I knew that much Italian, and the people told us it was all so very quick, so inconceivably quick. What the people could remember was the spring tide which came back. The sea threatened to engulf them. Yes. First, everything collapsed, and the people who survived heard more than they saw, because those who were *there* were all dead. There was no one left. The survivors were all far away. They heard the dreadful roar of the collapse, but all they could remember were the screams, how everyone yelled; for the sea became as high as houses. 'The sea is engulfing us!' And this tidal wave came up from the sea and those who were in its path became its victims. Yes. Dreadful. And the bad thing which followed was the terrible robbers and thieves. First one had to have one's life saved from the earthquake, and then from the spring tide, and then one lost it through these robber-bands which came.

There were three bands. They established themselves and took away everything, everything. They even undressed the dead and everything they had on them and they pillaged, because there were many treasures. There were all these palaces and everything. The churches, the wonderful churches with the many church ornaments. Just think of the gold alone. That must have attracted the entire population.

Well, that was Messina and no help could we give. So we went away from Messina, we went away from such tragedy. The weather was lovely. The heat had gone and the sea was blue and wonderful. It made an enormous impression, this lovely weather and the beaming

57

sun and those dreadful ruins. If it had been cloudy, that might have seemed better, but to look like that in the glaring sun.

Then we travelled for a short while up to Ancona. Ancona I can't remember. We must have been there only a short time. We got on to another ship and crossed over to Trieste. From Trieste we didn't go straight to Vienna; but to Umago, which is a tiny place on the sea at Istria. Today it has become a pretty place where one can go for the bathing season. But in those days, it was a place that no one went to. We went to Umago and I can still remember how the hedgehog ran about the room at night and we couldn't sleep, he smacked his lips so. He was looking for the cockroaches from the kitchen and whatever else ran about, and he collected them and smacked his lips, very loudly. So God knows we couldn't sleep, because of this smack, smack, smack. That's why I remember it so well. But he had beautiful big ears. The chameleon was quiet, but the hedgehog was impossible. Anyhow, the chameleon I took to Vienna and gave it to Professor Werner. When it was excited it got quite red. Just like a turkeycock. You know how the turkey's crop is? When it gets excited it blushes and the veins are blue. And it's the same with the chameleon. It changes colour and its eyes get to be bigger. And when it sleeps it can't close them completely, only half. A frightful beast. But the hedgehog I kept. In my house. Yes, smack, smack, of course all the time. But he perished then in the cellar at my parents'.

Happiness in Vienna

So here we are still at the time before 1913. So very long life is. And you want to rush me to Capri! Be a little patient with me. There are so many bad things to come. Let me go back again for a little time to Vienna, when I was naughty, yes, with my sin register, but there was so much happiness and no loneliness, never.

At the time it was very cheap to live. What impressed me greatly was that at the pork butcher's one could get scrump for nothing. Absolutely for nothing. On the day they made the scrump one could go there and was given paper bags full of scrump. And in the autumn there were Serbian prunes in the Naschmarkt on a Saturday; when the baskets were nearly empty you got the prunes, as a gift. In later life it was never like that any more, never more one got things for nothing.

Oh yes, once more it happened. Between the first and the second world war, they gave out wine in the autumn for nothing. They actually invited you. When we travelled through the Rhône valley, we got out and they invited us to the railway station to drink wine without paying. The barrels were still partly full, and they had to empty them of course to be able to get the new *raccolto* into them. And when we went from Lausanne through the Rhône valley wherever you stopped you could get free wine. Yes, it was friendly and amusing and kind, because later on they merely poured it all away. You know how it is. But in those days they were more hospitable and liked an enjoyable life. Why do people lack this thoughtfulness now? You think it was the prices? But there were prices then also, weren't there? In those days everything was cheaper, of course, but also much, much more cosy. There existed a natural *Freundlichkeit* in Austria too, which no more can you find. Today they are hard and selfish. When the sign of the *Heurigen* (new wine) was put up, everyone knew where to go. The populace, the labourers, packed their roast chicken in a bit of paper and went off to Grinzing; they weren't as poor as all that. On one side there was great poverty. But on the other the working classes could go out with the chicken. People were different. Much, much more friendly, and also much rougher, more primitive. The populace, the labourers, the simple people, the coachmen, a bit uncouth perhaps, but much more friendly than now. And this even though the division between the classes was very clear cut at that time. Nevertheless it evened up through this mutual friendliness.

The Crown Prince was the big love of the people, the people loved Rudolf, and were so shocked by the tragedy of Mayerling. It was the fault of the Emperor, because the Crown Princess Stephanie was always tittle-tattling to the Emperor, that Rudolf was deceiving her, and she felt neglected by him in every way. I often saw her walking in the Prater. In Vienna, she was unpopular, the whole of Vienna was on the Crown Prince's side.

And so the Crown Prince killed himself. Melancholy was the cause, discontent. The reason for his melancholia was that he couldn't get what he wanted. He tried to achieve a kind of freedom for Austria, and especially for Hungary he wanted it . . . but there were always opponents . . . And at the time he was in love with the girl who went with him into death. But even without Vetsera it would not have gone well with the Crown Prince, because the Emperor pushed him too far into the background. The whole of Vienna found this wrong. The opinion of the people about the suicide was: it serves the Emperor right, he asked for it.

Mama used to tell me how bad the Archdukes were even when the Emperor was there. It's a crying shame, the Court ladies said, even if they did hide smiles behind their fans, when the Archdukes ran around stark naked in the Hotel Sacher with only their sabres round them. Court gossip! Mama brought it home of course, but I was still too small then. One thing I remember well, and dreadful it was—the fire at the Ringtheater. My parents had seats in the first row of the gallery for the performance of a lady whose hair Mama dressed. Papa left the shop late, they were in a great hurry and they went up the Ringstrasse, so that they should still be on time, and when they were about to enter the Ringtheater, there were screams and the people stormed out. They were very lucky because they would have certainly perished. At the moment it was said—I don't know which Archduke reported this—that the fire brigade had saved nearly everyone. On the contrary nearly everyone was suffocated, hardly anyone got out . . .

Shirts for Gigi

In 1913 Papa had to sell the house in the Einsiedlergasse because he suffered from a heavy collar-bone fracture due to a fall, and following this a *paralysis agitans* which is also called Parkinson's Disease, and so the house was sold and we moved to Ober St Veit, in the country.

For Papa it was necessary to be out there in the country, it was quieter. I had a lovely room in which I

61

had nothing but animals, little dormice in cages, a guinea pig and a young hare. And that's where I took those animals I brought from Africa, the hedgehog which had not yet died, and the chameleon before I gave it to Professor Werner.

So this winter semester began, and in this semester . . . but I can remember nothing of it except how I sent Gigi three shirts, which I had made for him, beautiful shirts made of lawn, because as I told you, he was pretty low in spending-money down there . . . lovely white shirts. I don't know how I knew his collar size because I only saw him in his rowing shorts down in Positano, but the idea came to me that when he went down to Doctor Bauer to play the piano, he would wear one of my shirts . . . Doctor Bauer was from the Institute of Zoology in Naples, a German. With his wife and two children he was living in Positano and he had a beautiful grand piano and they had concerts in the evening. Ritzenfeld played . . . and Gigi in one of the white shirts.

And then the spring of 1914 came. In this spring of 1914 I travelled to Sorrento in March, and Gigi fetched me very nicely with a carnation in his buttonhole in a carriage and we drove over the Teresinella, which is this rise over the mountain from Sorrento to Positano. He still lived in Frieda's house. Ritzenfeld and Frieda had got themselves a permanent lodging. He let me have his room and he put up nearby somewhere. Behind the bed was a niche and there was a large snake in it, a house-adder, and he said, 'I'll bring a bowl of milk, because the snake is used to having its milk every morning.' I didn't much like a snake right by my bed, but it was the soul of goodness, and did me no harm. So there I was and there were concerts at Doctor Bauer's. Gigi had to listen to my papers as I was preparing for my finals, but we soon got bored with that. It was March and the weather was superb, and so we decided to take a little trip to Calabria. What a splendid time it was. *This* love affair went on. Yes, yes, this worked, this worked to order. I have told you, haven't I, he collected me with a carnation in his buttonhole!

So to Calabria and, to be sure, he had arranged with the fishermen that when they went again to Salerno and Paestum we could go with them. He in his rowing-vest and trousers, and me in a skirt and rowing-vest, and thank goodness I had sandals, he had none. They went barefoot in those days. On arrival in Paestum there was a storm, and to land the boat was difficult, and we had to leap into the surf, that's where my sandals came adrift, that didn't matter, half swimming, half crawling, we came to the shore, laughing too, you know how it is, and they took care of the boat.

That was towards midday, and in the afternoon we were on the plain which went from Acropoli to Paestum, and in this plain a thunderstorm started such as I have never lived through in the whole of my life. Because everything there is flat and swampy, we had to duck and lie in a ditch on the ground, for if we stood up we were afraid the lightning would strike us. It was all around, jumping like grasshoppers. But soon it was over, the whole thing was over in twenty minutes, but these twenty minutes were a big torment for me, I would never have thought that it could be so bad . . . After that the sun came out and we were soon dry. Then to Acropoli, a little place where you could eat, no, not in a pub, in a house, a large shop—in those days it was so—

in which you could buy everything, and you could also eat there, and there was even a room next door, and there we could sleep. Those sort of things no longer exist. It was very nice, although we broke the bed. It must have been a heap of rubbish.

When we came in to breakfast the peasants were horrified because Gigi ate four or five eggs at one sitting. They pointed at us with their fingers, and they said that he should buy me some wooden shoes. I can remember that one of the peasants took him aside and said: 'Get her some *zoccoli*' (wooden shoes).

One had to pay but what did one pay? So little it was, 5 centesimi, 1 soldo. For the bed which broke we had to pay 10 centesimi, 2 soldi. Acropoli was lovely, the Hohenstaufens had had a castle there, and the ruins of it were very well preserved. And from these we went to Ascea and Elea, which are excavation sites. It was March, but as lovely as in high summer, the peasants were so friendly, we used to have to sit down at noon, and they gave us wine and figs, such beautiful figs, and nuts, and we could eat as much as we wanted to, or were able. Then we came to Pisciotta, there is a beach there, one of those lovely, wonderfully long, long beaches. Pisciotta lies half-way above it and the beach went on and on, and when there were rocks jutting into the sea, we went over them, but if that was too difficult, we just swum round them. This was practical because Gigi could be completely naked and I only wore pants, but these dried again immediately afterwards.

No one bathed there. The beach was completely wild, deserted. Round the reef, then on again on the beach, endlessly to another sandbank, right to Pisciotta. Then we went up again to the railway and travelled down to Sapi and Paolo. There we paid, for the night (there was a tiny pub) with supper first, with wine, and breakfast, each of us paid fifteen lire—twice fifteen— thirty lire. That was practically nothing, as good as nothing. When we returned to Positano our own people didn't recognise us, neither Ritzenfeld, nor Frieda. We were like savages. It was lovely, very hot, and yet it was only March, but such a hot March.

Then I went away, I was already a little late for the summer semester. When the summer semester was ended in Vienna, towards the end of July, I again travelled down, by myself, straight from Vienna to Salerno.

War Declared

In July 1914, towards the end of July, I arrived in Salerno. Gigi fetched me, he came with the ship, there was still a ship which went Salerno-Positano-Capri-Naples. That exists no longer now as it did then. Everything has become worse, not better.

Now Gigi had a small house right up against the rocks, down in Positano, which he had rented; there was only one room and a tiny kitchen, all leaning up against the rock. That's what I moved into, when I arrived. Our friends were all there, we went bathing on the Arienzo beach, the whole lot of us, naked at night. Those last nights were wonderful, those July nights, and then suddenly the war broke out. One fine night there was a terrific uproar on the piazza in Positano, because someone had brought a paper from Naples. The bells tolled and they were all crying that war had broken out. The consternation was so great, as they had no conception what war was, there had never been a war, the last one in Europe had been the war of 1870, and that had not touched them, and eventually so greatly did they concern themselves that many cried out and beat themselves, and some even vomited, and some drank *vino* and sank under the tables.

We were horrified. Of course Doctor Bauer knew that I had to leave immediately. Gigi said that I had to go to Switzerland. And there was Professor Woltereck from Leipzig. He also said: 'Back!' He meant to Germany, of course, immediately, a declaration of war by Germany and Austria . . . we didn't understand a thing . . . It was all confusion like the days when the Saracens came.

During this last time in Positano, there lived old Gambarletta, he was an aged fisherman, and down on the beach he would tell us stories of the Saracens, how the women, and the men, everybody, fled to the mountains, up into the mountains of Monte Nocella. Everything of any value was walled up, and then they fled into the hills and waited. The young women though, they stayed because they liked to go away with the Saracens. The unmarried ones. They weren't at all eager to fly into the mountains. The Saracens remained a while, plundering, and went off again taking the girls with them, but what happened further to those girls we never discovered.

Those must have been summers, which Gambarletta told about, of immense heat such as we never experienced, and it appears that it was baking hot from February to November. New-born infants simply died, one had to take them to the cellars, they went through terrible heatwaves. It was a bad time, and there was always a certain fear in the people that the summer might again be frightful like in those days. When the first rains came in the autumn, in the middle of September, the whole population ran out dressed as they were or not dressed at all, and tore their clothing from their bodies, to let the rain bathe and cool them. If they were in a shop, or wherever else it might be, out they ran. It was a deliverance, in the sense that they needed really to feel the rain on them . . . I did not experience this, I only lived through the one summer, which was bone dry from February to September. But not the great heat.

On the day of the declaration of war, Gigi packed his painting things together. He painted such beautiful pictures, they all remained in the tiny house. He packed his painting things and I my suitcase with which I had arrived from Vienna. We set forth on our journey, and left everything else behind. The Bauers also left everything in their house, and all that too was lost. Ritzenfeld stayed at first—he didn't have to join up—only I, Gigi and Doctor Bauer, we went. We took a *carrozzella* (small carriage) and when we got to the Teresinella, one of the wheels was already broken, so we had to get out and we said, 'Oh dear, this will be a long war, this is bad.' We regarded it as a bad omen that the *carrozzella* broke down beneath us.

We came to Naples, from Naples to Rome, and in Rome we just about caught the last train to Germany and Switzerland. I can still remember how we ran and ran after the last train. The flags waved, they yelled after us, the Italians wished us all the best as we were leaving. It came so suddenly, this declaration of war, in one day everyone had to leave. Doctor Bauer got out in Innsbruck and changed trains and got to Germany and

we went to Switzerland to Gigi's in Basel. His parents
were in Basel. They had a house there. And me he
brought into a side street and found me lodgings and
then later presented me to his Mama.

Marrying Gigi

At the first encounter, he introduced me quite naturally. I had been in Capri, accidentally, he said; we had
been travelling with Doctor Bauer and he had to go on
to Germany, so everything was decent and above-board
by even the most conventional standards, and in the
side street I was staying with a lady, who gave me a
room. As usual, I was a naughty girl, but on this occasion
the alibi was as convincing as it was mendacious.

And then the telegrams began to arrive from Vienna,
'Return immediately'. Whatever had got into me, my
parents wanted to know, not to take the train from
Rome through to Vienna instead of taking the train for
Switzerland, and I think I justified myself by saying
that that train was the only one that came at the moment, and it seemed safer, and in short, there I was.
Gigi had immediately to join up as a conscript. He was
only just twenty, he had to report in Basel and was then
ordered to Lucerne to the training centre . . . I, of
course, instead of going straight to Vienna, travelled
with him to Lucerne and lived there for a few weeks and
took a room in the house of a certain Mrs Kaufmann.

We met every evening. Every evening I stood outside the barracks and waited till he came out. Apart
from that I looked at Lucerne, I walked around and
prepared myself as best I could. You see I had to take

68

my orals for the final. So here I was in Lucerne, and then, curiously, we went down the Bahnhofstrasse, and he goes into a shop and he says, now we are going to buy each other engagement rings. We hadn't agreed to this at all and I said that I didn't want to get married. But we bought the rings then, and as my parents got more and more pressing, I went off to Vienna, sad because of all the changes that were forcing us apart. Then I felt happy with my ring. Gigi had to go and report to the border, for frontier duty when the training period was over, and I travelled to Vienna and a hundred thousand questions they asked me then, poum! poum! poum! Why had I remained so long in Switzerland? Why this, why that? And I told them nothing of all this then.

I took off the ring. It was prudent. I wished no emotional disturbance at this time, and I went and prepared for my orals, and I went to the last lectures. It was autumn 1914 (in 1915 I got my degree). And now, of course, I bullied Gigi and wrote and wrote, and he got leave after doing two months' frontier duty, two months' leave. And for this leave, as I had insisted, he came to Vienna and I took him to the sister of Frieda Abeles, to Dela Abeles, out there in Doebling, and she had quite a nice room, and there were two small single rooms below her, and she rented them to us, and he came and took up residence. I lied like a trooper then and said, 'I shan't be home for one week because I must be in hospital, to do the midder and that's why I must live in the hospital.'

So I was on duty during the day, and sometimes during the night I was in hospital, but at other times I didn't of course go home, but went out to Doebling.

The single room. And it was very jolly at Abeles' house. In the evening we went up to the Tuerken-schanzpark, there were roundabouts, and there were Hungarians, I remember, or gypsies. They told fortunes. One told my fortune in the courtyard of the General Hospital, the Allgemeine Krankenhaus, just before I took an examination, and I only wanted to know if I was going to pass the examination, but she wasn't at all interested in that, instead she said, 'You have a long life, many loving and beautiful children; but you have no luck.' She spoke the truth, you see. That was in the year '14, before the finals, which I took. I wanted to know nothing, but she told me this! A long life, there you are! But no luck—that too she said.

I did not take Gigi to see my parents. I knew what there would be—poum! poum! poum! I was nearly thirty—what difference would that make?—poum! poum! poum! I explained, and it really was true in a sort of way, that I needed a room near the hospital, because I had to study very hard and prepare for my finals so that I could get a good degree and be able to go to all lectures. So I rented a room in the Schwarzspanierstrasse for the remaining time before my finals.

I was of course not alone, because Gigi came, from Doebling, and one day Mama came too. So I admitted I had taken this room and I admitted everything. But she already knew, one of the women who cleaned up must have told her, because I was questioned and all details came out. Lies I cannot tell, real hard lies with no bit of truth in them, I have no use for them, and I just said, yes, I had met him, and Mama said we knew something must be up, the letters and so on. And then there was a dreadful row, my God! This is no honourable relationship, and this is terrible, and poum! poum! poum! They wrote immediately to Gigi's parents in Basel and proposed a meeting. All this in a tempest.

I thought, just see how it is, this Civic Virtue! It is the same loud smacking of lips like with my hedgehog, but without the good reason of wanting to eat cockroaches. Yes, I was angry, I too smacked my lips, I did not accept these old parental insults, I was *stuffata*. These narrow views make me quite ill in my bowels.

Well, those from Basel, my mother-in-law to be and my father-in-law to be, came in due course and arranged among themselves the financial aspect, and to put it mildly, marriage, immediate marriage. I had money, and so had he, they had seen to that, and they told us we had to get married and have the banns called in Basel and also in Vienna at the town hall, and I still remember how cross we both were because we had neither of us ever thought of it as wrong. And we were right, and all of them absurd like primitive tribes. The difference is: in an 'honourable' relationship you live apart, first you are a *fiancée*, then a bride and you have no sexual dealings, and the other thing is 'dishonourable'.

When it was discovered that we had two single rooms in Doebling and that in the Schwarzspanierstrasse he had been always seen with me, then poor Dela Abeles got an earful from my Mama. And my Papa and my Mama, before Gigi and I left for Switzerland, said, 'Our consent you don't have; you are entering on this marriage without our consent.' They said that from the very beginning, in which they

71

were, of course, proved right, that this was a marriage which couldn't possibly work. They said, 'He is seven years younger than you, a painter, and an unreliable person.' And those in Basel had to agree with this. Financially it worked because those in Basel said that he didn't have to live only by his painting, there was quite some money, and he was their only son. The father was a director of the State railways, they were very well-to-do people. So that's how it went, and Gigi and I travelled to Basel, and we were married, at the registry office in Basel. I did not want to become a Protestant and so we had no other choice. So that at least was a favour I could do my parents, when I said, 'No, no, I will not take another religion, I will remain a Catholic.'

They would not come to Basel, and after the registry office we didn't celebrate the wedding with Gigi's parents but travelled out to Landhaus-am-Rhein, which is upstream, a small place, wonderful, and this was during the cherry-blossom time and all the trees were in bloom. And there was an inn, and this is still called Landhaus-am-Rhein and there we celebrated our honeymoon in this Landhaus. It wasn't really a honeymoon, but it was technically a honeymoon. I have told you he was so beautiful a man.

Because of a Simple Foetus . . .

Of course we didn't stay long. Gigi had acquired a painting commission through Doctor Bauer, who had been transferred to Koenigsberg during his military service, to make a portrait of Hindenburg. He was a good portrait-painter was Gigi. And so we travelled to Koenigsberg.

We went to Koenigsberg via Munich. It was lovely in Munich still. We were in a little place near the city where they breed trout and char, and there we had a second honeymoon, much more beautiful than in the Landhaus, and then another again in Munich, and then we went up to Koenigsberg and rented a room somewhere near the zoo. Friday was the day when the meat-eating animals were not fed, and the lions roared, but apart from that it was lovely, and in Koenigsberg I immediately went to help (for it was in wartime) in the hospital. I had got my degree a month before we left Vienna. It was a lovely graduation ceremony with Tandler and Reinhold.

Gigi didn't come to the graduation, but Mama did (Papa was paralysed). It was only for the wedding that they refused their blessing. The degree was for General Practice. In Koenigsberg, I went to work for Professor Winter in the Gynaecological and Midwifery Department, as assistant *interne* and I gave the anaesthetics at the operations. One always gives this job to beginners, and I was really quite efficient as anaesthetist. One day while giving an anaesthetic I collapsed and became unconscious, and there was Doctor Bentin, and he said afterwards (he called me Liesl): 'What's the matter, Liesl, what's up?' I told him I had got to feeling deadly sick when I did the anaesthetic, and he said, 'I am going to examine you.' 'No, no,' I said, 'there is nothing wrong.' Well, he examines me, and I am in my fifth month of pregnancy.

I had noticed nothing. You see, as a young girl, my period would sometimes come and sometimes wouldn't come. I was without for months on end, and I was always a little thin and anaemic. I only noticed that in Munich the beer didn't taste quite right, but I didn't think of this. Doctor Bentin said: 'You are finished with anaesthesia.' It was summer, so he said it would be better to go to the sea. Gigi had earned quite a lot with his portraits, and so we went to the Kurische Haff, the Kurische Nehring, with beautiful sand-dunes and beach: there I was very well. Gigi was so pleased, he was like a fool with pleasure, and his parents and my parents were immediately informed, and then the communications came from my parents, yes, we will forgive everything, only you must not stay longer in Koenigsberg, we will rent for you a flat with a studio for your husband in Doebling. So it was. Because of a simple foetus, everything was to be lovely in the garden. They did not give their blessing for the marriage, but now they were full of joy. And then we travelled to Vienna where we lived in the Cottage district, high up on the Peter Jordan Strasse in a studio with a room.

You want to know about Hindenburg, but I did not meet him, only Gigi did. On the one side he described him as a rude one and on the other as a very good man. He was offensive, Prussian, but, hidden deep down, very kind. Gigi also painted a portrait of Ludendorff, but that was later. It was in the summer he painted Hindenburg, the summer of the battles of the Masurian Lakes . . . We celebrated the battles in Koenigsberg, the big victory of Tannenberg. We were at that time in Koenigsberg at the Blutgericht, which was a subterranean drinking place. There were many of those East Prussians who at other times never opened their mouths, and there they yelled and roared and boozed and we were half-seas over, both of us in the Blutgericht.

Peter Jordan Strasse: that was very beautiful in the autumn, and the Tuerkenschanzpark was wonderful. And just at Christmas, the 24th December, Gigi had to bring me to the hospital to have the baby, right on Christmas Eve into the maternity hospital, where there followed a big fuss, of course. The professors all knew me there, Professor Thaler and all. 'So now here you are in a different capacity,' because I had always been a little cheeky. 'Now you are a bit woozy.' And poor Thaler had to leave his Christmas tree in the middle of the night. It was a difficult birth, the child was in danger and I had a forceps delivery. When I awoke out of the anaesthetic, I saw him, lobster-red, and he had a lot of black hair, the little boy. I didn't remain there long. Poor Mama had brought a goose for Christmas, which swam about in the bathtub, it should have been killed at the very last moment for a goodly Christmas dinner, and I had to make such a situation, upsetting all plans and keeping that goose swimming. She never thought that I would have a little boy, because Papa had always said, 'She'll never manage to make a boy,' because I had always been a pathetic little thing, such a small one. He was called Ludwig Philip Moor, but afterwards when I went to Capri he would be always Ludovico.

On the fifth day when I couldn't even stand, I wanted to leave, so Thaler said: 'If she insists that she doesn't want to stay we'll let her leave. I'll take the stitches out at home in the Peter Jordan Strasse.' It was lovely, at home. Gigi had arranged the room with the view so beautifully; marvellous flowers, red roses, it was winter, I can't think where he managed to get hold of them. I was *completely* happy. Mama came, a big to-do, to and fro, to and fro. And we lived in the Peter Jordan Strasse, he as painter, and that's where his models came —he always had flirtations with the models.

I didn't mind that. I had told my parents in advance that this didn't mean anything. They had said in those days: 'You'll see, this won't work,' but despite that . . . He was so very sweet to me it really didn't matter, it was quite unimportant. This I tell you is the truth. You do not believe me because you think I have always been a jealous one. But it was not so. This is the truth.

A friend of mine, a certain Gundi Patai, who was the daughter of Mayor Patai of Vienna, came to visit me with her small child, and I wheeled the small Ludovico in his pram into the Tuerkenschanzpark. We were very, very happy. Truly, for me that time was perfect happiness, even though it was the bad wartime. If we hadn't had parcels every three weeks we would have starved. It was possible to send a beautiful parcel from Switzerland, coffee and ham and sugar and all kinds of things. The grandparents sent them. Because in Vienna there was only a kind of turnip. Bread was made of *mais* (sweet corn), and it was stretched out with Danube sand, awful, it fell apart, so your mouth was full of grit.

I fed the child myself, but in order to get milk for me my husband got rid of everything, even his last pair of trousers. He didn't *sell*, it was barter. He gave them away to the milkman in the Peter Jordan Strasse. Money no longer had any value, so when he had a pair of trousers of his own, or when they sent an old pair of trousers from my father-in-law in Switzerland, then one could get the litre of milk which by law one was entitled to, but which you could only get from the milkman if you slipped him something. And that was Christmas 1915.

So now we are in the spring of 1916. The child's milk came from Switzerland in tins, and ordinary milk from the milkman to whom we gave the presents. To fetch coal we had to go to the railway station early in the morning. Soup we could make from clover, which wasn't at all bad, and there were those turnip things and everything somehow went all right. At the confectioners one could buy a kind of chocolate cake (but it was not chocolate, what it was I don't know to this day, some kind of black flour), and there was *mais* fat which came from the Balkans, a yellow fat which looked like yellow seeds, and always the turnips, and the clover, we had nothing else.

We were still there when the Emperor died. I was standing in the Mariahilfer Strasse when the funeral went by. At such a bad time it made an enormous impression on me, an enormous sadness. In that broken time of war, one suddenly forgave him everything. Because of his age and the misfortune of his son and his wife, one forgave him, and one could see the whole tragedy in a terrible sense striking all the world. As a child I had seen him in a march past of our schools in the Ringstrasse, in the year of his Jubilee, and that's when we at school marched right by his tent and I saw him quite close to, and when the Czar of all the Russias was here he drove by in the carriage, and again I saw him quite clearly. The Empress I also saw close to in Schoenbrunn, at the back in the locked part of the castle, through the fence, yes. And when I ran in the morning across the Ringstrasse to the University, I often saw the Emperor drive by in the early morning coming from Schoenbrunn on the way to the Burghof to work. And all the people would stand absolutely still on the Mariahilfer Strasse, and one could see his white plumes from afar, and that's when I very often saw him: an old man, who stood very upright but showed no goodness in his face. An apathetic face, a face which had lost interest. But the Empress, when I saw her, was exactly as one imagined a beautiful good fairy. I could not detect any suffering in her face. The expression was beautiful, just as if she loved all her subjects and understood their lives.

It was not long after the funeral that Papa died. And after his death we immediately left Vienna.

He was old, I think in his seventy-sixth year, when he died. He was of course affected by Parkinson's Disease and by the deprivations of the war, although Mama did everything for his nourishment, but nutrition was no longer the same; above all there was no milk, and no meat. The illness made everything more rapid. So those in Switzerland now began to urge us and said that my Mama should not remain here either, and so we went to Switzerland.

It wasn't quite as simple as all that then, because it was during the war, and it was hard to get entry and exit permits. My husband had to sit in a valley in the Tyrol in quarantine, and we two (the boy was then not even a year old) we could travel on, and there in the Tyrol Gigi sat, and only joined us ten days later. We went to Seelisberg on the Vierwaldstattersee, and there we rented a small villa, the Villa Flora. It was lovely in that villa together with my Mama. Now all was well between Mama and Gigi. When the child arrived, and she looked after it, then everything was all right.

We were told very emphatically at the border not to start eating immediately because there were many deaths from sudden overeating, and that was quite right. We hadn't eaten all that much at the frontier, and in Seelisberg we weren't used to it. We were famished, emaciated, skin and bone, and now suddenly there was the heavy Swiss milk and butter, but it was very good all the same. It was beautiful in Seelisberg, and we went with the lovely pram into the woods. Only when the *Foehn* blew, it wasn't so lovely, because then the Villa Flora shook, the neighbouring roofs were stripped of tiles; one couldn't go into the wood because the branches and tree-trunks flew into one's face, the *Foehn* was dreaded. So we spent the whole winter of 1917–18 in Seelisberg, and then . . . strange . . . but so life is . . . you must not be angry with me . . . I am a bad one, but God made me so. Him you must blame if you have to blame.

The Russian Lover

Into the Grand Hotel came a cellist, a very famous man by name of Hermann, with his two daughters, and practised to get ready for an American tour. Hermann was a German, and broke his journey in Switzerland, and there was an affair between Gigi and Maja, one of the daughters. She played the cello, a huge woman. And on my side, I met in Seelisberg a Russian tenor by name of Wolkow . . . and that was also an affair. What an affair. Like Hell it was! He was a wild one, I tell you, and when Russians are like that, you get to be afraid of them.

My goodness! What went on in that wood! Never was I a goody-goody, you have understood this, I had

a lot behind me, but this was unheard of, really unheard of. It pleased him also, and the beauty of the thing
was that, when we were in the wood, he would sing
arias in between, and then he would start making love
all over again, and I would say, 'No. Not again. Not till
you sing me another aria,' and so again there was more
singing and more love. He was like a *mitraillette* that
man! It was all pop! pop! pop! A woman cannot know
what love is like if she has not made love with a Russian.

The good Gigi he went God knows where with his
Maja. Why should I care? He was not in the woods,
that was sure. But there I was with this Wolkow. How
strange that once all these things happened. So long
ago. It is very bad to be old and not to go into the woods
any more. Sometimes I dream at night that I make
love. But that is not good. It is terrible.

As for Gigi and Maja . . . at that time it didn't matter
to me at all. Only later it mattered. I had Wolkow and I
was really quite used to Gigi going with his models. So
I thought, this Maja, she's no model but a cellist, and
anyway she's going to America, and so I didn't worry
too much.

But it was only for a short time, that affair in the
woods with Wolkow. He had to go back to his country.
I was sad, how sad I was. Sad like Hell. I said, 'I will
come with you to the frontier,' and I went just like
that, leaving Mama and my child and Gigi, not saying a
word. We took the train to the frontier and at the frontier there was a little *albergo* and we stayed the night
there, and we made love, but I do not think he sang
any arias. And next day he took the train to Italy and I
took the train back to Seelisberg. I was not frightened.

I did not think anything would happen. After all Gigi
had his Maja.

But when the train came to Seelisberg Gigi was there
on the platform, and of course there too was the station-
master and the porter, and Gigi took my arm—he was
very polite when he greeted me and we went to the
hotel and suddenly there in our room he took a stick
and he beat me so hard I nearly died. I kept very quiet,
but the child Ludovico cried and my Mama knocked
on the door and I thought he would kill me, but I kept
quiet because after all it was right that he beat me. I
even began to love him again because he was a man and
he did right to beat me. But what he did after, that was
not right.

Don Domenico and the Devil

The Armistice came. We were still in Seelisberg, but
Mama was pressing to return to Vienna, because she
must have her flat back. And because of the money, the
devaluation, she lost even that. We had this war loan,
which it transpired was only a piece of paper, so she had
to go to Vienna and we went to Italy.

We packed up the small Ludovico, and we moved
from Seelisberg, with a trunk as large as a coffin, and
we went down direct to Sorrento. Maja had gone to the
United States and Wolkow to Russia where there was
the revolution and I never heard of him again, but that
Maja affair—that was not over. My God, no!

We arrived with the immense trunk, and it was
loaded on to a large landau and this drove over the
Teresinella with us to the Hotel Manna in Positano.
All the world had changed with this bloody war, Gigi

and I had changed, but Positano was just the same—only the evenings on the terrace with Frieda Abeles and her friend and Gigi on his guitar—that was not there any more. Why do the good things go when the bad things always come back, even at night in dreams?

The first day we went down to the beach. Ludovico was two and a half years old and still wore dresses and he went straight into the sea, as though there were no sea, no fear, I can still see it before my eyes. I was so scared, the little dress billowed, and then we fetched him back and showed him that opposite were islands, the islands of Galli, and we explained this to him, and he was interested. He was interested in everything. During the night it was frightful in the hotel. Bedbugs there were, and when we got on to the beach the next morning, he pointed to the islands and said: 'There, there the Winzeln,' which was a union of *Wanzen* and *Inseln* (bugs and islands).

We stayed on in Positano. There were other Italians from the North of Italy with whom Gigi became fast friends immediately, and there was a priest, Don Domenico, who became his greatest friend. This Don Domenico, he was a priest, the best priest imaginable, but not a puritanical priest. That certainly not. He liked girls and he liked boys, whichever came his way. I can remember he always carried figs, dried figs and nuts and almonds in the pocket of his what-do-you-call-it—soutane?—and he would tell the little boys—and the little girls—'Come here and feel in my pocket. You will find something there for you.' And of course there were the figs, and what does it matter if their fingers touched something else there too? It did no harm. He was a very good, a really good man.

At this time there was also an episode which the writer Andres used in his tales of Positano. Where the road from Amalfi leads to Positano there is a large water-trough on the road, where the coachmen water their horses. Now this Don Domenico one evening laid himself completely naked into this horse-trough, and in the evening in the twilight horses came harnessed to a *carrozzella*. So when they stopped in order to drink, and saw this naked man, they shied, and the *carrozzella* rolled backwards. There was a dreadful precipice behind and there could have been an accident. The people all thought that it was the Devil in the horse-trough. So Don Domenico ran like Hell and no one pursued him.

Of course Don Domenico didn't mean to frighten the horses, but he wanted to scare someone else who always went by there to fill his barrels with water, him he wanted to scare because he had something against him, forgetting that at that time the horses would come to the trough.

He was really a delectable priest. He went to people, and if ever any butter or something lay about, he would pinch it. He never used it for himself, he took it to the poor. He also took this and that from me; this and that disappeared. So he simply said, 'I took it with me. I brought it to those down there, their need is greater than yours.'

There was a hunchback in Positano then who always visited Gigi. He was of a patrician family, very well-to-do, who owned large dyeworks, silk dyeworks. I can remember how Don Domenico (he was fat and thick-set and at the same time very agile, he could jump), how he danced with the hunchback Clavel one night, lifting his soutane so that one could see his naked legs, while Gigi played the piano. Those were good times. Not like the old time, but good all the same.

Now we had left the Hotel Manna. We had a house, a lovely house with a balcony and a terrace, which we had rented, and Don Domenico came up there, and one day when the *Tramontana* was blowing, all the crockery, the plates, were thrown in one swoop over the sill of the terrace into the street below. That's how strong the wind was. If one was on any of the flights of steps in Positano and the *Tramontana* came, not even a grown-up could go on, you had to sit down; it came in thrusts. When one blow came you had to wait, and then move forward a little before the next thrust. Rather like the *Bora* in Trieste, where people have to hang on to ropes. That's how it is in Positano when the *Tramontana* begins. So there we were in Positano, and that's how it was.

After the first war quite a few Swiss people came to Positano, and oh yes, Doctor Bauer also came back with his family. He found his house as good as empty and moved down to the beach at Tonillo into a tiny house, because he had lost everything. He returned, and Frieda Abeles came too, and so did Ritzenfeld, but then she picked up a Jew, a certain Wolf, and they opened a kind of Co-op where one could buy cheap foodstuffs . . . It wasn't a great success and only lasted a short time, but that's what they started in Positano. It was all very different after the war. There was Doctor Bauer and Frieda Abeles and Gigi and me and Ritzenfeld, but nothing seemed the same as it had been.

I did not practise as a doctor, only as a mother and a housewife. Next to us in the villa there lived a certain Arlotta, an Italian. He had a very beautiful wife, a

Russian with wonderful blonde hair, blonde plaits, and a son whose name was Valoddia and a daughter whose name was Pucci. They became great friends with Gigi, and Gigi painted the Russian woman, and it was no flirtation because she was most carefully guarded by the good Arlotta. I kept my eye, too, on him, just a little. I am only mentioning this thing with the Russian lady, because later (I was at the time pregnant with my daughter, and the Russian had this wonderful blonde hair), everyone said it was because I had been so impressed with this Russian woman that I had such a blonde daughter, because the boy, Ludovico, was very dark like his father, and she had gold-blonde wonderful hair.

You must not complain to me that I do not say always one thing after another. The memory goes this way and then that way. It is not like soldiers marching all in order. So now it is that I want to tell you a little more about Don Domenico because I have told you only the funny things about him. That horse-trough and the figs and dancing with the hunchback. For those reasons the Bishop did not like him and at last he was sent away, but he was a good priest, not a rotten one at all, and he was loved. When it came to dying, the whole of Positano called for him. He was the best father-confessor at the end, and it was with him one travelled best into the next world. It was he alone who was fetched to the dying, no other one would do for the people. Because he was so delightful, so funny, the people had to die with Don Domenico. Everyone, be it man or woman, he was their confessor at the end.

Gigi and Maja

I have told you how it was that Wolkow went away for ever to that damned revolution, but I was not finished with Maja, the bitch. It was not enough to have been beaten till I nearly died. In Positano I had always to go to the post office to fetch the letters, and there I noticed there were letters to Gigi from Switzerland all the time and then I discovered they were from Maja. That made no difference when I told Gigi I knew. Gigi sent me just the same to fetch the letters of Maja, and that was more cruel than the beating he gave me after Wolkow. That I deserved—poum! poum! finished, but this I did not deserve, to fetch him the letters Maja had written. One day I opened one, and in it she wrote and fixed a rendezvous with Gigi in Cremona. She had to go there about some violin, and she wrote to him that he must come to Cremona, and she will then take him to America, she was that crazy about Gigi. That is when I began to be terribly hurt, and Gigi one day he said then: 'Now you must accept this. I am going to Cremona and I will see Maja there, you can have anything you want from my parents for you and the boy, they will go on helping you, to look after you. I want to go with her to America.' She had bewitched him completely.

I can remember how I went weeping to Don Domenico, and how he talked to Gigi telling him he shouldn't do this, that this was fearful to destroy such a happy marriage. And then one day we were on the beach with people from Basel, an architect who built houses and wanted to build new villages. His name was Hauser, I think, and Gigi had the habit of throwing big stones, not into the sea, but at a man made from stone, and I know Hauser was sitting next to me when a huge stone missed my head by inches as it went by, and Hauser yelled: 'For God's sake, you could have killed her!'

Gigi didn't do it on purpose, yet I know I was absolutely terrified, and we were walking home and I said, 'You should have been more careful. You are going away, but do you know that I am having another child? I didn't want to tell you . . . But there has been nothing doing for two months, and sometimes I feel very sick. I am having a baby.'

'What?' he said. 'You are having a child, well then, the thing with Maja is no good. I can't do that sort of thing,' and when we got home he sat down and wrote to Maja in Cremona and told her she should go to America by herself, he had a wife with a boy, who was again pregnant, and he would not leave her. There was a big to-do, Don Domenico was very happy. Gigi said: 'I am no scoundrel, no, I don't do things like that.' And I wondered, did it matter what he did or did not do? It was a little desolate, yes, certainly.

Then we went . . . In Positano, one couldn't stay in this condition, everything was very primitive, there wasn't even a hospital, and thus we went away and stayed with the in-laws in Basel, and it was the time of the carnival, and despite my in-laws' advice I went to the Baseler Carnival, in this very huge fat condition, and right on the first Sunday after I arrived I had to go into the Maternity Hospital in Basel, and this little girl came. It was a normal birth this time, not like the first one. It was difficult, but no surgical intervention.

So now we lived with his parents in Basel, we were married people with children . . . This little daughter, she was called Julia, Giulietta, and when I went home with the little child to the in-laws Ludovico was very unhappy about this sister. He was five years old then and didn't want a sister. We only noticed this when she was taken to the bedroom to sleep. There were very lovely pink ribbons on her cradle, and when we went up from the dining-room, Ludovico had cut all the ribbons off, tore them to shreds, there wasn't a single ribbon left.

The birth was in March 1921, and after three weeks we left Basel and went directly to Capri, to Anacapri.

PART

2

Typhoid in Capri

This was how it it came about that we went to Capri. A chance. Always there were these chances in my life. Ritzenfeld finds his Jewess and brings her to Positano, and his Jewess is Frieda, so I go with Alfi to Positano on the way to Africa, and there is Gigi in his rowing shorts. So it was with Capri—chance—it was only a visit this time, but in the end I was to stay there for more than forty years.

You see, Gigi had an acquaintance, Italo Tavolato, who lived in Anacapri. In Florence they saw a good deal of each other. It was Italo Tavolato who found him a house in Anacapri, and we lived there in this house, directly on the Piazza Caprile, that still stands.

It was a very lovely July, a wonderful July. We always went to the lighthouse to bathe, me carrying the little one . . . and then I got typhoid, a very bad case of typhoid. Apparently it came from the Pozzo water and the diluted milk and the heat. There were a lot of cases, and Professor Rispoli was called in. My husband worked down at Lady Gordon Lennox's as a painter of frescoes, and she said she would get one of the grey sisters from the Villa Helios to be my nurse, and so it was. The grey sister came and looked after me. In those days having a case of typhoid was not as it is now, when one has all these antibiotics. In those days one was simply given a little quinine, three-quarters of a litre of milk a day, and mineral water . . . Yes, and some hope too. But it was the nursing which was the most important. One was given wet compresses against the high fever, damp cold compresses all around the body; that was still the old way of dealing with typhoid and fever.

It was dreadful. During the day Gigi worked at Lady Lennox's and in the night he came. I was very brave about the typhoid, said the nurse, but the child cried all the time, and so for the child we took a wet-nurse, Annunciatina, a peasant, and she still had her own baby. All the same Giulietta cried a lot during the night, and Gigi was angry, and I remember how the sister was flabbergasted, I can still see how it was in my fever with the sister in hot pursuit of Gigi, 'Mr Moor, Mr Moor what are you doing?' He couldn't stand the yelling another moment, and so he put the child into the garden and the sister ran after him . . .

For three weeks I was between life and death. Next door two died and in the whole of Anacapri there were at least ten deaths. It wasn't very pleasant. And the thing was this. After three weeks I was getting better and then Gigi got typhoid! But his was an easy case.

We then moved away from there into the Villa Boffe, a very nice little house facing the sea with a beautiful terrace, so that we had a little change of air. And then we went back to Positano. I know that this journey was a trip which no one else would have done . . . It was a very rough sea, with Ludovico and the baby, and we had this *forno di campagna*, which is a small cooking stove, and the chamber-pot, and everything fell into the water. There wasn't a quay, and the ship had to wait outside the harbour, and there was the *Tramontana* blowing, and we had to disembark and the chamber-pot and everything fell into the water, but they fished the pot out just before it sank. And thus we arrived in Positano. We lived in a different house, where once the post office had been, and the people we knew came to us, and also Don Domenico, who came immediately.

A Naval Officer Called Tutino

I lived in Positano with my husband and two children and made the acquaintance—and now comes the really serious affair—of an engineer and naval officer, a certain Beniamino Tutino, who lived with his mother and his sisters. They had a villa in Positano, and I got to know him on my trips with the pram, because I always wheeled it into the valley of Ajenzo, and so I met him. He always walked there, and he always carried a novel by D'Annunzio, and when I walked past, he would follow me and push the pram. He was very good about pushing the pram and started immediately to read me D'Annunzio. This repeated itself in the afternoons, because my husband painted round about that time. It was the reason we had come to Positano in the first place, because he had been commissioned by the municipality, by a family who had returned from America, to paint an altar picture in the church, a picture for one of the side altars, San Nicola. It is still there in the cathedral of Positano, the first picture on the left side of the gangway. I am no longer sure, but I think St Nicholas is freeing a child out of a wine-barrel (no, no, it was not propaganda for teetotalism!).

This was the picture he was painting, and so he was busy during the daytime. And every afternoon, I walked in the valley of Ajenzo with the children and Tutino. And so it developed into a friendship, and in

93

the evening we went to fetch the milk, from a peasant, who lived there. The hill where she lived was called Minchia Pendente. That is really rude. It means the hanging tail, but we only knew that later. When my poor child Ludovico also used these rude words which he had heard, like *strunzo* (well, that means shit), it took quite a long time to persuade him that one did not say them. So there we went walking with the perambulator, always we went to fetch the milk; we were walking once, also with the child, when I fell down a rock and had internal injuries, injuries to the spine, one can still see this on the X-rays. So many walks there were, so many words and so much D'Annunzio, and all the time Gigi was painting St Nicholas, and for his part he fell in love with a German *Fräulein*, a certain Katessky . . .

He did not know about Tutino then, but he knew that I went for walks, perhaps he thought, 'There she is in the woods again like with the Russian Wolkow,' and when one evening I wasn't home he waited for me and beat me thoroughly, and what was worse, once on the terrace he threw knives at me so that the neighbours had to be called. He must have thought things out for himself. Why would I go to this rather distant valley of Ajenzo, and every afternoon at that? But this kind of thing he allowed freely to himself. Well, he was a painter and so it is with painters.

You ask me how one can make love in the open air with two children. Why not? Ludovico would run to the beach or to the waterfall, there is a very lovely waterfall, and the little one was only a tot. Safe in the perambulator.

When Gigi beat me I had this feeling in myself, well,

you have earned this. On the other hand I wanted to know, was Gigi now so good himself? After all he had this thing going with the German girl, he was not a conjugal model. We were wrong, both of us, but what reason can there be for a one-sided fidelity with its terrible illness of jealousy?

My Mama had remained in Vienna, she had a flat there, and the government wanted to put in strangers—it was the time when no flat was allowed to remain empty, when everything was commandeered, and nobody was allowed to have a vacant room. So Mama had tenants put into the flat at Ober St Veit and was very unhappy about this. Then she wrote her son-in-law, Gigi, that he should go to her in Vienna. Those people —there was something about payment, some kind of legal row, and she asked, as an old woman, that her son-in-law should come and help her against the tenants. And Gigi went to Vienna and I remained alone in Positano with the two children. And Tutino had to report for duty, he had to serve again as naval officer, he had only been on leave, and he had to join a ship in Brindisi. He said I should go with him and I took the children to the wet-nurse in Capri, who had once fed Giulietta, and I went with him to Brindisi.

I locked the flat and the children were with the nurse in Capri, and there I was in Brindisi, until after a few weeks I could no longer bear it without the children, and one evening I took a fast train to Salerno and thence on to Capri and Positano and took the children back to Brindisi, and I still remember, there was no room for them, so they were on four mattresses and a chair in the dining-room. Thus I accommodated them in a primitive kind of way. Next thing Tutino was ordered from

Brindisi to Taranto, and I also went with the children to Taranto, and then again he was stationed in Naples. And in Naples we wanted of course to remain together and so we took a room for me and the children in Naples on the Mergellina directly on the sea, and he remained in the Navy in Naples.

Ludovico at that time became really naughty. (It was not that he was jealous of Tutino. They got on very fine.) He squabbled with his sister, he hurt her. The children were not well behaved, they smashed the mirror of the woman where we were lodgers and everything became a little out of hand. Ludovico rushed about with the Neapolitan boys, he didn't always want to stay with his little sister. So I engaged a German *Fraulein* because things had got out of control, but soon the *Fraulein* had to leave, and then there came from Basel a relative, a cousin. But really she was a damned spy.

A Daughter of the Devil

It was said she was going to visit Rome, but she ferreted me out in Naples. I don't think it was at Gigi's instigation, as he was with my mother in Vienna, but at the instigation of the parents-in-law who didn't know why I should suddenly be in Naples. Always these suspicions. Why should people be so suspicious? And yet I must admit there were always these transgressions too, so they were right in their way.

How did she find me? I suppose I must certainly have written to my husband that I was in Naples, because I was still in correspondence with him. So to Naples she came to spy, and shortly after there arrived letters from Basel, and they spoke about Ludovico who would shortly be seven years old, and would need a school. The grandparents insisted they did not want him to go to a school in Naples, but I was to send the boy to the grandmother in Basel. Well, I did that, and of course I should not have done it. Even Tutino said, 'Don't do this, keep the child here. We will manage it somehow.' For there were even a few classes in German, but I thought to myself that perhaps that wasn't the right thing, not because of the schooling, but because he was always in the streets.

When he was gone to Basel to those Swiss there were no rude words, no transgressions, no one spoke of a hanging tail. But I suffered terribly. I dissolved into tears, and I suffered for a whole five years. Now I reproach myself, but this does not make it any better, all these reproaches for always obeying self-indulgence even at such a cost of suffering. Was the cousin not wrong too, what she did? She only came once to the flat, she just blew in, and how she could have found out about these things, as she didn't speak much Italian, I cannot imagine, but anyhow she must have informed herself, and then written. The inquisitive woman is not the mother but the daughter of the Devil, and always, too, a virgin. Who would make love with the daughter of the Devil? A dry bitch who could not bear happiness. She met Tutino, in the street, not in my room. But nevertheless, she grasped at once that something was going on and that's when the offers about the child's schooling were made. Then I had to travel with Tutino —he was off again down to Sicily. At first we had been for a while up at Posilippo, which is by Naples, and had a very nice flat in the house of a Russian woman, really very pleasant with a kitchen and all.

Tutino was a good-looking Italian, not as tall as Gigi and not nearly as beautiful, no comparison, but lovely curly hair, and by physical nature a little weak; he needed a lot of vacations and leaves because of his health, and he was perhaps a melancholy one, always reading D'Annunzio. He did not like being in the Navy. He was younger than me, six years younger. They were all younger, I had only young ones. Even as a young girl, they were all younger. It was not good. If I had got the right husband long ago, instead of Gigi, perhaps everything would have turned out in more constructive ways. Though not so interesting. That may be true.

It was a bohemian life with Gigi, and with Tutino too, in the sense that one was always travelling, because he was always being ordered from one ship to another. We travelled everywhere, to Sicilian harbours, to Gaeta and Formia, and I followed him with the small Giulietta wherever he went. I could not go on his ship for he was on a battleship. I stayed on land, and when he was finished in the evening he came on shore.

An Agreement with Gigi

Once I went to Vienna with Giulietta. Gigi no longer lived with Mama, but with Zuzzi (what a name!). He had rented a studio not far from Mama's flat, namely in Unter St Veit. And as a model he had this Viennese, a tiny delicate creature, he could have packed her in a suitcase, in a large one. He even did this once for a joke. I would have posted her to Siberia, the bitch! He, of course, also had visits from previous models, a large girl from Bohemia, an enormous female. I don't know her name now. She had been a model whom he had painted previously, but she kept on coming, and also a colleague of mine, a young woman I knew in my youth, who was also in Vienna; he also got going with her. Oh, he was well taken care of. You need not feel any sorrow for Gigi.

I met Gigi immediately when I arrived. Mama knew all about these models, although he never brought them to her house, but she knew all right what happened in the studio . . . My Mama was very fond of Gigi, she liked him better than she did me, her only child, and always agreed with him, and when he came to Vienna to get her out of the flat trouble, that boosted him very high in her estimation.

Somehow we came to an agreement, and it was arranged as follows—we even put it in writing—that I could remain in Italy and he would live here, and the child Ludovico would stay with his parents and Giulietta with me, and we would live apart, but in case I should have a child by Tutino, then I would have to tell him. Yes, that's what we had written down. I gave my consent, to tell him if a child came. Otherwise I could live for my part how I wanted, and he for his how he wanted.

You ask if Zuzzi was not afraid when this wife suddenly turned up all the way from Italy with a little girl. But no, it was all friendly, we had the most enormous fun together. On my part just a pang of jealousy when he put her in the suitcase.

All my husband's mistresses were my friends, he on the other hand, towards Tutino never . . . In Positano he could stand him on sufferance only, he never gave me to understand that he knew I was having an affair;

he just behaved as though denying it all the time. I, on the other hand, never had anything against these girls right from the beginning of the marriage. Well, why should I have something against them when I myself...?

Then I went back down to Italy, because Tutino had written incendiary letters. I must come at once. He couldn't bear it alone another moment... He was very much in love, and I too, I suppose, but I have the impression he must have been more in love than I was. Even his mother wrote to me that I shouldn't make him bear this, her son was dying of grief. If I wanted, we could get married. But Gigi and I had agreed: I didn't want marriage, and he didn't want to marry either. It was very, very important to him that I did not marry anyone else. I will tell you about this later, and about the crying . . .

The Torments of Jealousy

I went down to Tutino again, because of the passionate letters, and because I had decided to take the Italian diploma (medicine) and it was very convenient because Tutino was at the Military Academy at Livorno. So I travelled with the little Giulietta also to Livorno, and there we lived together, because he was not on a ship but at the Academy (he had to do a course or something as lieutenant). Pisa was close by, and so one day I went to Pisa and enquired about the qualifications needed for an endorsement of my Vienna diploma in Italy. I was informed that there was no longer any such authority and that I would have to take the finals in Italian all over again. I was a foreigner, and as a doctor I would have to be able to speak the language perfectly, so that the people could understand me, and also because of wider medical understanding with my colleagues. All the final orals would have to be passed in Italian, and this was to be in Pisa, because it was near Livorno.

Then I procured the set books in Italian and in Pisa I met a colleague, a medical man, a certain Venanzio Loggi. He was a friend, really just a friend. He offered to help me and let me know in Livorno what it was I still had to catch up with; he also helped me with the papers and the whole arrangements for the examinations. And from time to time I went from Livorno to Pisa in order to prepare myself, which then provoked the most fiendish scenes of jealousy with Tutino, and that was dreadful.

Gigi used to throw knives at me, like a variety act, and nearly killed me, but Tutino, he only tormented me, he talked and tormented me, and followed me to Pisa and made a scene to Loggi, who assured him a hundred times that we were engaged in more serious affairs without time or thought of nonsense, he regarded it as his duty to help a colleague, and that apart from that there was nothing personal in it. And Tutino, of course, didn't believe him and begged me stupidly on his knees that I should not go on studying further, that this was not at all necessary, that we would anyhow soon get married and so on and so forth. But this I would not agree to and would not be dissuaded.

I had met Loggi when I was enquiring of the Professor of Gynaecology, whose name was Professor Gentile, about the examinations. Loggi happened to be there, and the Professor said: 'Why don't you explain to our colleague about the whole method of our examinations, and give her a bit of a hand?'

Loggi was very nice. I liked him a lot. It wasn't a sexual thing, it was an extremely good friendship. He made an impression on me, he was a tall North Italian, a blond bear of a man, and it pleased me greatly that he should have helped me like that. Apart from that there was nothing doing with him. When he escorted me to my train to Livorno, we'd go to drink another espresso in a bar, but that was about all, yet despite this, Tutino was madly jealous. From autumn till the summer, nine months, I worked for my degree in Italian, and then I passed all the examinations, quite a few of them with distinction, nearly all *cum laude*, and so got my doctor's diploma in Pisa.

And there I can remember exactly, while they were all congratulating me, also the Professor who *was* a little interested in me (in Pisa it is customary to put a laurel-wreath on one's head, which is not the custom with us in Vienna), Tutino arrived. He had taken time off only to take me straight home; there should have been a bit of a party that evening, but no, he said, now you've got your degree, that's enough.

Professor Gentile was very kind and said that if I wanted to practise anywhere, if he could be of any help to me, he would do it. That was in 1922.

Gigi sent me for my graduation my first beautiful real silk dress, embroidered, dark blue with tartan trimmings, it really was a lovely dress. He had bought it for me in Vienna and he sent it me packed very badly, and when the parcel arrived one might have thought it was just a bundle, and Tutino hadn't thought of anything like that, because he didn't want the graduation. How angry he was. It was the last straw that Gigi should have sent me the dress. Tutino was posted to Gaeta, so

I had also to go with him to Gaeta, and because I wanted to have Ludovico come to Gaeta, that made him more angry still—well—imagine! But I had begged my parents-in-law that, when once I had my Italian doctorate, Ludovico, whom I hadn't seen all those years, would be brought to the frontier, to pass his school holidays, the summer holidays, with me in Italy, and the mother-in-law had agreed to this.

In Gaeta I declared to Tutino that now I was going to go to the frontier, I *must* see my son again, 'You can no longer say anything against this,' (nothing would have made any difference). A foul journey it was, from Gaeta in various trains as it's not very direct, and I went to the frontier at Chiasso, and there sat my mother-in-law, most unfriendly, and said: 'I trust you will take care of the boy.' So I said: 'Of course, yes, and Giulietta is also down in Gaeta.' To this she said: 'And when the holidays are over, he'll have to come back here, and you must not again send him, like the last time from Naples, with complete strangers, and he only seven years old,' (because when I had sent him from Naples, I had entrusted him to a Swiss woman who got out before him, and the boy thus arrived alone in Basel). Ludovico's journey must have been all of five years ago, and so when she said this I said, 'I promise. As I collect him, so I will return him.' We only spoke those few words together. It was the frontier, she stood on one side and I on the other, because I didn't cross over to the Swiss side. She could just hand the boy over with his little case.

So we travelled down to Gaeta, and things really started all over again. Now Tutino was jealous of the boy. Ludovico had brought his butterfly net and his specimen-box, and we went to Lerice, the lovely beach of Gaeta, and Tutino had always to go back to his Academy, and when he came to join us on Saturday or Sunday, then he was jealous of the boy, as well as of me. 'A woman with children all alone on the beach, an Italian will surely strike up an acquaintance,' so he thought, and so of course they did. Tutino knew this from his own experience. Had not he done it himself long ago in Positano when he read D'Annunzio and pushed the pram for me?

Oh, no longer to have anything to do with an Italian, I thought. It was a real torment, this constant jealousy. And Ludovico said, 'Why not leave him, he is always so nasty with you?' He didn't, of course, really understand all of this, he only saw that there were these continual scenes, so he would ask, 'What on earth have you done now?' And I would answer, 'Well, we mustn't go to the beach quite so much,' and then he would say, 'Why not?'

There was no trouble with Ludovico. We got on famously. We made excursions to a tower with the little one, and she was also very happy. Ludovico was very friendly now with the little one. He helped her with her swimming, all through the summer holidays, three or four weeks, and then I had to take him back.

So Strange is Life

I don't know if I should tell you this. When I travelled back with the children to Chiasso, to the frontier, we first went to Formia, and in Formia I met a man on the beach. It was only quite superficial, he showed us the beach at Serapi, and so I made a date with him. I can't tell you what his name was, it was only a very little affair. He was a bear of a man, an Italian. He explained to me on the beach at Serapi the whirlpools, the sudden deep patches in the sea where you could drown even if you could swim, because the current pulled you down, and he explained the whole area to me. I had nothing really sexual with him, we just exchanged that odd little kiss.

Then in Rome where I went to take the direct train to Switzerland, and also show Ludovico St Peter's, there was another man. He was an Air Force lieutenant. I still have his photograph. We met in the train to Rome, and he interested me quite a bit. We were only a very short time in Rome, and then he had to rejoin his squadron, but with him, well, there *was* something . . .

Then I travelled with the children to the frontier and handed the boy to his grandmother who was waiting for me with fierce eyes. She wasn't at all nice, much crosser, and I handed Ludovico over and went, feeling so sad and hurt, with Giulietta down to Sicily because Tutino's job was finished in Gaeta. I took the boat from Naples to Palermo, and in Palermo there was Tutino again, who had taken a room for me and the little one in the same hotel where I had stayed with Tolleg. So strange is life.

The Birth of Andrea

That was in August, not a good time. It was terribly hot and I always felt dreadfully sick, which I didn't much care for, until I noticed—'Hello, now you are pregnant by Tutino!' I couldn't say this with complete certainty . . . The father must be either the naval lieutenant Tutino, or the Air Force lieutenant, so any-

way the father stayed in the armed forces . . . It wasn't
Gigi's, that was sure, because he was in Vienna, and on
the frontier there was only my mother-in-law. This was
most important when the divorce came about, because
I couldn't pretend this other child was my husband's,
although the odd thing was that everyone said the child
so resembled my other children, that no one would ever
have known that the child wasn't Gigi's . . . he seemed
more Swiss than Italian.

I told Tutino and I said, 'I don't want it.' He said he
was delighted and he wanted it, but me—no. I wasn't at
all pleased. First because I felt sick and with the others I
never felt sick this way. (When I think what a terrible
thing was to happen later, this is both biologically and
psychologically interesting.) Only with the first one was
I a little sick with the anaesthetic. I felt wretched and it
was very hot.

It was the last naval station where I was with Tutino,
and then he went back to Positano and actually in
Positano below his parents' house he had a small house
in the garden, and we lived there, but without the complete consent of his mother who was not very happy
about it. She wanted us to marry, but now there was no
longer any talk of this, and she was not at all pleased. I
went to live with him in this little house only because I
still had to take the State examination in Naples. I had
the doctorate from Pisa, but in Italy after the doctorate,
in order to practise, one had to take the State examination, and thus I had to go to Naples. I was in fact in my
sixth month of pregnancy . . . There was little Giulietta,
Ludovico was in Basel, and I travelled to Naples for
the State exam twice on different days, for surgery and
internal medicine. Everything went well with the ex-

amination, then back to Positano. But things were bad there.

As to the pregnancy, we had decided (because I had had such a difficult time with my first one, and also the second one in Basel hadn't been exactly easy) to go to Naples. It would have been difficult to leave Positano at the very last moment, so we went for a week to Pozzuoli, which is in the vicinity of Naples, and now things suddenly began to happen, and one evening we went to the Swiss Hospital in Naples, and there came a boy, Andrea. This was in the year 1926, in the spring, on April 2nd, and on the fifth day I started a horrid puerperal fever, with septicaemia, then nephritis. I nearly died.

It doesn't sound possible, does it, even in 1926 and under the most primitive conditions? It wouldn't have happened in a Swiss hospital at this time, to almost lose one's life. It was not the fault of the Chief, Doctor Sutter, a Swiss; he of course did all he could, he gave me intravenous injections, and it ended with kidney complications, and I left too early, because I was scared. I had to go to the town hall in Chiaia in Naples to register the date of the birth and I gave the baby my maiden name Andrea *Klaeser*. I couldn't give him the name of Moor, naturally, because he was not my husband's. One can't do things like that, for there I was in Naples with Tutino. No one knew in Vienna or in Switzerland of this birth, that I had nearly died. Tutino was delighted, but he was like a frightened little rabbit. The whole thing was most embarrassing to him, above all because I nearly died and he felt the responsibility.

From Naples, of course, we returned to Positano, and in the house where we lived it was most primitive.

I was so very ill, and had these constant haemorrhages from the kidneys. It was wretched in those days. I breast-fed the baby, and soon noticed that that would not do, because the poor little one got thinner and thinner. The milk was affected by the fever. So we looked around, and found two wet-nurses, one from Montepertuso, and one from Montepecello, farmers' wives, who came and fed him alternately. The child was debilitated, but he regained some of his weight through the good breast-milk.

Tutino's mother who lived up there in the big house with the same garden paid no attention whatsoever to me. Except once she sent down the local doctor because I was so bad. She never came down herself, and didn't bother with me. And so, off my own bat, I found a German girl who was living in Positano, and begged her to help me a little with the house, and to help me with Giulietta and the baby. I was forty. It wasn't very good (no one has sympathy for a woman of forty who is *disgraziata*), and one day there was a squabble, actually because of this German girl, who came to the big house and begged they should do a little more for me, and there was a fight, and I packed my trunk and moved into a room with my two children, near the Chiesa Nuova.

A Divorce

Of course Tutino made a terrific fuss, but I simply couldn't bear it another minute and on impulse I wrote my friend, Dela Abeles, the sister of Frieda. I wrote that the child wasn't well anyhow and I must come to Vienna, because I must tell my husband. The child was at the time seven months old. I wrote in order to help myself, because I didn't dare to go to my mother with the baby, although Gigi no longer lived with my mother, but in his own studio. (The Zuzzi who was packed in a suitcase was not there any more, but already there was another one!)

I wrote to Dela, I'm coming, and actually went. Dela Abeles came to fetch me at the Sudbahnhof and we went straight with the baby to the Reichsanstalt, somewhere out of Vienna, but Giulietta was with me, and I took her to my Mama. Then I confessed to her, that I had gone first to the Reichsanstalt and dumped a baby there, another grandchild . . .

She was very, very angry. It was quite terrible. 'Thank God, you did that. I would have been too ashamed in front of all the people. This can't go on. Your husband, he comes here, yes, every day. We have our meals together and all . . . and you turn up with another child!' I thought this performance would never stop. It was all very bad for me. She said, 'I don't even want to look at it, this brat,' and I said, 'You don't have to look at it, I don't want you to look at it!' Then I went away and the child was in the Reichsanstalt and was being well looked after, and it had a wet-nurse there also, and then they weaned it, so that I could take it away with me again.

That was the thing with Mama. Gigi's people, of course, said, 'This can't go on, you must apply for a divorce. When she has a child of another, this can't go on. The other two children are financially endangered, and so is the inheritance.' (In those days they had money, you see.) 'You must apply for a divorce.' And I said to my husband, 'A divorce. All right. I want to have the divorce in my disfavour, because this is true that I have the child of another,' and although he had also been unfaithful, I still begged to have it this way. 'You do the divorce, but the child, Giulietta, stays with me. I admit my culpability, that I am the guilty party, but I demand my daughter for myself.' She was then between six and seven years old, in her seventh year, a beautiful child.

The divorce proceedings took place in Basel, and later Ludovico, my son, who became a lawyer, explained to me that it was a thing which was not in order, because of course one couldn't give a completely guilty party the custody of a child. I didn't have to go to Basel, they fixed it all, and then they informed me that I was divorced and that through my guilt any right to any inheritance was null and void . . .

Yes, they were very clever, the good Swiss, the whole divorce was only about money really, not on moral grounds, and I was forbidden to marry for a year. I was not to marry Tutino ever, this was stipulated, but Giulietta I was allowed to keep. Is not this a disgusting kind of barter? Yes, and for Giulietta I was to get alimony of one hundred francs. In those days one hundred Swiss francs was something. One hundred Swiss francs per month I was to have, which I of course never received but that is another thing . . . I expected and wanted nothing of those people.

And then there was this business with my Mama. Mama was of course extremely vexed with Gigi because of the divorce, and said they should not have done that.

Of course in those days divorces were very rare and she agreed that this was only a financial thing, and was very unhappy with it. She also demanded back the beautiful big diamond ring which she had given Gigi as a wedding present. He gave it back and all my jewellery, and with this I bought my medical paraphernalia, instruments, etc., and returned with the two children, Giulietta and Andrea, back to Tutino. He was in Rome now in the Admiralty. He had taken a room and bought a giant bed.

There I came to the Monte Sacro—Citta Giardino it's now called. The little Giulietta I sent to school in Monte Sacro and I went in Rome to Professor Ascoli. I knew that till the money started to arrive from Switzerland I would have nothing, and I got work translating from English for Italian newspapers, and from Italian papers, where he wrote articles, I translated into English for him, so that he could publish them in English papers.

Tutino said we should at last get married, which I didn't want, because I no longer liked him. I only wanted the children. I stopped liking him when I had Andrea. Well—I have to tell you that—I was never very faithful, but Tutino, yes, he was good. Anyway, I didn't want to marry him, I didn't say no immediately, but I said: 'Later . . . later.' Always I said to him 'Later' (like the Spaniards—yes?—*mañana, mañana*). Then Giulietta got a very heavy pneumonia, she brought that back from school, from drinking cold water after her gymnastic class, and when the summer started, I said the child needs to recuperate and I am going to Capri, to Anacapri.

PART

3

To Anacapri

It was 1926, and I travelled with the two children to Anacapri. I wanted to stay there for the holidays, and I wanted also to look round Anacapri, to see if I could earn something there. Those articles for Professor Ascoli in Rome, that was too little. I had brought my medical paraphernalia from Vienna, the medical diploma I had, I was allowed to practise, so I thought I could manage it.

I arrived in Capri as poor as a beggar. My mother in Vienna only had her old age pension, and that was a few *groschen*, from which she couldn't even live, but she had taken in a lodger in Ober St Veit, and with that together with the old age pension, she could just manage, but she could give no help. All our money was gone.

So I arrived in Capri with a dress on me and nothing else, not even underwear. Oh yes, I had on me a vest and pants, but apart from that, nothing. And the two children—they went barefoot. It was pretty bad, and yet in a way it was good. There are those long steep steps they call Phoenician which go from San Michele in Anacapri to the Marina Grande. In a bus now less than a quarter of an hour, but by those steps? Half an hour and it seemed nothing, with Giulietta on my back, to go and bathe at Tiberio after work was finished. She had no shoes, but I had to have them for those steps. Running up and down it was hard, but it was fine like Hell all the same. Life was hard but it was happy. I am one of those who like running. The worst of old age is the walking, so few steps this way and that.

Those in Switzerland they no longer wanted to know anything about me—otherwise why would they have insisted on the divorce? They had agreed on the one hundred Swiss francs for the child, but these only came for the first few months, and afterwards nothing more came.

Tutino remained in Rome at first, then he became ill and suffered. He always had things wrong with his intestines and with his bladder; he was always ailing, and perhaps as a naval lieutenant he may have overworked, because he always went on studying, he was an engineer by profession.

He remained in Rome and then he went to Positano to his mother. When I was at Anacapri, he came over to visit me and he came as he used to do and moved in with me, and we lived together as though nothing had happened, although I knew in my innermost self I didn't want to marry him, so I didn't want to accept anything either . . . And those in Switzerland sent me nothing, and I wanted to take nothing from Tutino, so I was forced to take up my profession. And that is what I did, and it worked like a clockwork, I at once had clients. After one and a half months I gave up the flat in Rome and the giant bed and the few bits we had there . . . I had them sent and we lived at Teresina Cataneo's in Anacapri.

It was during this time that there came the attack by those men at Anacapri which I have told already. The morning after that attack, I went to the police and asked if they could protect me, or if I would have to send to my consulate. In any case, I was not going to be attacked again and especially in such a murderous fashion, and the Maresciallo had them brought in, and they of course arrived with a wonderful alibi firmly worked out, where they had been on that particular evening, so that it would have been impossible that it should or could have been them.

And then the Maresciallo said: Good! If in the next few days, if even the least little thing were to happen to me, they would be clapped into jail. And he warned them and also me he warned and said: 'You see, the whole family of these people is now infuriated. They have lost their child, and all this talk means that the family is dishonoured because it was consumption.' And not only had they lied, but also they had brought false testimony, and only God knew where they had been, so at present he was unable to take action.

And there was the wife of one of them, and she yelled in my face that I was telling a lie, I was a German *strega*, and uninhibited as I was—I know how this can be a bad thing—I slapped her face in the full view of the police, and I shouldn't have done this. And then she said she would of course make a law case out of it because of these doings.

Now the Maresciallo, who saw that I had got myself into the wrong because I didn't want her to lie, and that I couldn't control myself, said, 'You know what you should do, as they are now so incensed, why not go for a few days, for a week, to Sorrento, until this excitement is smoothed over, because I believe you have done a lot of good here, and on the whole the people are on your side and all this is only of the moment?' And that I then did.

When I returned from Sorrento, the whole house was full of flowers and baskets of fruit. All the people came and said they wanted me and I was not to go away; it had been so dreadful when I had been away in Sorrento, and they even got so far as to make the woman come and apologise and say that she would not make a lawsuit against me, and I bought her some material for a beautiful dress and everything ended well.

So I went on practising, and had a lot more patients. I worked extremely hard, but I didn't earn very much, those whom I knew to be not very well off I refused to let them pay me. They loved me a little perhaps in their way, because they could see that I was for the poor.

The Cerios

Edwin Cerio, who had once been Mayor in Capri, belonged to the most esteemed family in Capri. Edwin had a villa in Anacapri, and he discovered through one of the maids that there was this foreigner who practised, and that I had carried out an operation on a hand, and that all people called me in. So when he had bronchitis he told the maid: 'Well, fetch me this foreign woman, this *dottoressa*;' and then he became my protector because he found out about everything, and because he was very satisfied with me in my capacity as doctor.

He also introduced his brother Giorgio who had married Mabel, an American. And then Arturo Cerio, the elder brother of Edwin, fell seriously ill. He always suffered from severe asthma, and otherwise was in bad health, so that his brother Giorgio and Mabel then begged me I should go with him for a cure to Bad Reichenhall in Germany. This I did and I tended him. Giulietta was placed with the German sisters down in Capri, and Andrea stayed with Tutino. He took him to his mother in Positano. The cure did Arturo a lot of good, and he gave me in gratitude five free days in order to go to Switzerland to see my son, Ludovico. He was at the Gymnasium (a public-school boy) and the five days were lovely and amusing, and we walked along the Rhine, and then we went back from Bad Reichenhall with Arturo; from Genoa to Naples by ship, so fine it was.

What a famous strange family were the Cerios. Anyone in the world who has heard of Capri has heard of them. Edwin had been for a time Mayor of Capri, and did a great deal for Capri and had made himself liked and disliked as it is in these cases. Giorgio had been married before, his wife died suddenly, Jenny had been her name, and he had a large tomb put up for her. Giorgio was a doctor, he took after his father Ignazio, who had also been a doctor, a most beloved doctor, a scholar and archaeologist and mineralogist and all kinds of learned things. The piazza—that famous piazza—is called Piazza Cerio. It was called so after Ignazio Cerio, who was beloved by rich and poor, and then there were his sons. As I was saying, there was Edwin, actually a naval engineer, who wrote many books about Capri. Giorgio was also a doctor, but he didn't practise, and the third was Arturo, who was ailing.

They were always at daggers drawn, so that it was not a good relationship. Giorgio had married the rich American and thus acquired riches, whereas the Cerios on the whole were not rich. Ignazio had his family house in Capri, but what else he had didn't amount to wealth; the beautiful property came from his wife.

After the death of Giorgio, everything was divided

up. The property was distributed; Arturo died, Edwin outlived him, but he didn't inherit all, because Giorgio had had a child from a very simple Anacaprese, who was first taken away to France, and then he confessed this to his wife Mabel who took the child as her own, when it was six years old. She paid the mother for it, so that she would give up all claims to it, and would let her have this little girl who was now regarded as her own child. She had no children. I knew the child. She was very gifted, she learnt to speak English very quickly, although at first she had spoken only the dialect from up there in Anacapri with her mother. And she learnt good manners quite naturally and immediately became a young lady. She was remembered in the will, for when Giorgio died, and Mabel died also, Amabel was left the fine property on the Marina Piccola. The house in Capri Amabel also got, and Edwin Cerio was left with the palazzo, the original house on the piazza, and other fine villas in Via Tragara. The best, the Certosella, he bestowed on his daughter, Laetitia, a very lovely person, and she now works hard to maintain a cultural centre and a museum in the palazzo where she also arranges fine concerts, art exhibitions, lectures and so on.

Arturo Cerio was very nice, but so old, and always ailing, it was sad to be with him. When we had been a short six months away we returned to Capri, and when winter became spring, he fell ill with a heavy attack of pneumonia and he died, poor him. That was in 1930 I think. I received a little more money to be sure, because I remained the last nights to attend him.

A Vile Coward, a Creep

From my savings I was able to buy a house in Anacapri. It was a very old house in Caprile, one of the oldest houses, where everyone seemed to have lived at least once during their lifetime. A very old house, quite a ruin. For instance the staircase that went up was only a hill, the rooms were there, but everything was in this ruined condition. It was managed by a certain Damiano, and it belonged to three brothers who had emigrated to America, and had left it to Damiano; and so he was able to sell me the house and I paid 12,000 lire for it, which was even for those days, very, very cheap. But for me, who in those days was paid ten lire for a patient in the surgery, and twenty lire for a visit, it was after all a small fortune. The amount to pay for the house I had, but not the sum to pay the notary, that I didn't have.

And I didn't have it because at exactly this moment I had my savings in the bank, 7,000 lire in the Banca Astarita, on the advice of the marvellous Edwin and Giorgio Cerio, for when I had said in those days that I wanted to invest my money safely, they both laughed and said: 'The Dottoressa, she needs the Bank of England. For her princely 7,000 lire, she needs the Bank of England!' Well, anyway the bank went bankrupt the year after this, and my 7,000 lire went bang with it, and the interest too. Their investments they had taken out in time, of course. Oh yes, they were clever, the Cerios. Like Hell! This was only the first piece of 'good advice' of the Cerios.

So I lost my money, and for me this was a fortune, if one reckons it in ten and twenty lire, and so it came I was only able to pay for the house but not for the notary.

So I had to sell my beautiful microscope. I actually sold it to a colleague, who always came over from Naples, he was a specialist in gynaecology, Cicaglione. And he and I got together and opened up a surgery in Capri on condition that he could come over once a week to do his consultations there, but that otherwise it would belong to me. At the same time I also bought the necessary surgery furniture, also a gynaecological couch, and what else one needed in a surgery, and this was in Capri, quite near the Piazza Via Lungani.

So you think now all is well with the Dottoressa. There she is, even if the bank has stolen her money, with a consulting room down in Capri and her ruin up in Anacapri, and a fine partner. Fine partner like Hell! He was a small *vigliaccone* of an Italian! How do you say *vigliaccone*? Vile coward, creep. You will excuse this word, because usually I am fond of Italians, but this one, he was pushing, he wanted me to make love with him and I didn't want to. For God's sake, I couldn't stand him. And then I discovered that he used his surgery hours as a gynaecologist to do abortions. I was not involved in this, but when I discovered what was up, I not only found this uncomfortable as a deception but I became full of fear, because it was quite forbidden, and at this time the law was very strict. So one day I said to him: 'Now you get out and do not any more return.' Then he became abusive and made threats, and I said: 'You do not threaten me: I threaten you with a visit to the *Questura*.' So yes, then he took a boat and did not come back. All the same I kept my surgery. It was not easy at first but it got better. Many of the girls asked me for abortions, yes, but this I told them they must do in Naples. On Capri it is always *troppo amore*—too much making love. This is natural, but when you are paying these consequences . . . that is not so good. They say it is the air of Capri, especially when the wild herbs are out in the spring on Monte Solaro, and they say too it is something in the volcanic soil. Edwin Cerio called his book *That Capri Air*. Poor air that has to take so much blame.

It was a very bad time also with Tutino, because he of course had been against it from the beginning, that I should share this surgery with this Cicaglione. Jealousy again. He knew nothing about the other thing, that abortions had been performed. He was no longer a young boy, but Italians are like that. He was about thirty-eight then, and me—I don't know—more than forty. Age makes no difference in those things. Who am I to talk who was always a jealous one too? Men, they all rage, and women, they rage worse, much worse.

So I just said to him, '*You* didn't find me a surgery, so what do you want?' Financially I had no help from him because he was no longer with the Navy. His health was too poor and he was dependent on his mother. And although they were wealthy—there was only the mother now—not a soldo came to help me. Later his sister opened a *pensione* in Positano. Later still, an uncle made him a loan with which he bought some land on Capri on which he built a house. It is true, he helped me with the renovation and repair of my ruin, but I had to pay all the workmen, he only helped as engineer with the plans and the ordering, how they had to do it, and how they could finish it off, and so on.

They were doing it for one and a half to two years until it was converted. Then, with the house at last finished, Tutino was still half in Positano and half at

Anacapri. I had so much work then in Capri, many calls because of the surgery and I began getting all the patients. It was a time of unceasing work.

Grand Patients and Poor People

That was also the time the Harold Trowers were there. He wrote several books, Trower did, about Capri. He was what they called a British consular agent and he wrote about Capri even before the time of Norman Douglas. He had a beautiful villa in Cesina on Capri, and he was a patient and I cured him. He was not at all admired by Norman Douglas, nor by Compton Mackenzie who both lived there part of the time.

Men like him were my grand patients, but many, many more were poor people. Once I remember I was called to the lighthouse. There are always three families in the lighthouse, and two men were taken ill. It should have been the municipal doctor who undertook this matter, but he happened not to be there, and so they called me to come. And so down there I went and cured them. A throat infection, as I remember, and I stayed down there for two days. Nobody knew however that I had gone to the lighthouse, and so they looked for me everywhere, in the whole of Capri, and then it was discovered that I had stayed down there, and of course it was interpreted . . . because the wives were not there you see, and I was alone with three men, and of course there was one of them who was not ill at all and was capable of anything, thank God! It was one of those things, everyone who knew me teased me, saying I had disappeared without trace and hidden in the lighthouse. I was mercilessly teased.

You know what sort of people are these Caprese? I will tell you something. In the beginning, when I practised in Capri, there was a priest at the Marina Grande, Don Salvator, who went to the sick as male nurse. He was interested in nursing people, he helped them, and when I ordered injections he gave them. He did all these sort of things for the sick, and so when they took against me and I had for a time to disappear to Sorrento, one part of the doctors was against him, and on the Marina Grande where it goes up towards the Metropole, they caught him and they hurled him down.

He did not die, it was glossed over, although he also knew the people who did it, nothing happened to them ... They were so evil—there is no other word. And I, who in Anacapri had helped everyone, they attacked, but me they didn't catch. I tell this only to show what the people were like then. Now they are no longer like that, no longer so wild.

Another thing to show you how people were in those days. Once I saved my colleague, Doctor Procillo's life, because we together were with a patient with diphtheria, a child. Procillo was the doctor in charge, and he called me in as his assistant, and he made a larynx—an intubation: one puts a rubber tube into the larynx—so that the child could breathe. The larynx was covered with the diphtheria membrane, and the child died as he made the incision, a sudden heart-failure, and the peasant concerned, the father of the child, pulled out a knife and jumped on my colleague, and I leapt into the fray, hanging like Hell with all my strength on to the wrist near the knife, so he could duck out of the door. The man didn't pull his knife on me because the doctor in charge had been the other, and there was despair in his anger, and I tried to reach him with gentle words and in this I succeeded to calm him a little. My colleague knew his whole life long that I had saved his life.

Well, I had a great deal to do, and I could not be often at home, so for the children I had a girl, once this one and then another one. You know how this is in Capri with the servants. They were all such young things, fourteen to sixteen years old. They came into the house and helped. They were half children themselves, and there they were one day, and not the next, and then again they would steal, and had to be sent away. And in the evening there was never anyone, because at night they had to go home to their parents, they were only allowed to help during the day.

So the thing was that Edwin Cerio liked my Giulietta, and my friends brought home to me I shouldn't be so naive, that something might happen to the child, she was now thirteen years old . . . It seemed to me at first just one of those sick specimens of local malice which grow like a virus on that island. I did not believe any of it. They said I should . . . At the time I had not yet had a love affair with Edwin, that was later but not at this time. Perhaps later I would have been suspicious. You know a man better when you have made love with him . . . Well, to keep the peace for those concerned, and also among those who only wished to create mischief, I sent the child to Switzerland to a horticultural school, and she remained in the horticultural school, and learnt gardening. This school was in Brienz, on the Thunersee. Did she go willingly? Well, when one transplants someone from Capri into Switzerland, it is not so good, but it was not too painful, for Giulietta loved gardens.

The mother-in-law paid for all this. It came about in this way because I had frequently complained I had not received the allowance laid down for the child. As you know, I had only received this in the very first year, right at the beginning, and they were very wealthy, those in Switzerland and I had to work for everything. Thus Giulietta went to Switzerland and the little Andrea stayed with me and went to school.

He was a very lively child, he rose up as energetic as the sun and he shone all day. Yes, a kind of radiance; he was a child who was very much loved, everyone loved him, the old and the young. They always looked for him and wanted him near, then they were happy: he was a kind of *talismano*.

I have to append this: Ludovico had been a model boy. When he was still in Positano, as well as when he was in the Gymnasium, he was always top of his class, as well as afterwards at university. He studied law, and in scarcely three and a half years he was through with his studies and able to take his doctorate, and later the advocacy. Yes, he was a very brilliant boy, but Andrea— Andrea had this radiance. He went first to primary school in Anacapri and then to the Gymnasium down in Capri at the Certosa with the monks. That's how it was with my children ... Now come the men. Does that make the Dottoressa a wicked woman? It is normal, is it not? I was not an old fat thing like I am now.

A Handful of Men

First, Tutino always came a little to Anacapri, but he wasn't all that good. There always were the same scenes, the same yelling. '*Me ne vado!*' I'm off! Everyone will be able to confirm this, and then he would go to Positano and after a few days he would turn up again. And again: '*Me ne vado!*' *Oufa! Questi Italiani!*

He was ashamed? Huh! Just as though he had never gone away! And he justified his returning: 'I had to see my boy, didn't I?' And then when he was there, he would perhaps look over Andrea's prep; went for walks with him. He looked after him a little, that is true. And then he would always come up with this thing: he wanted to recognise him as his son, he didn't want any longer that he should be known as '*figlio sconosciuto*'—an illegitimate child.

And then there was a teacher. Yes, he was quite nice, and he took an interest in Andrea when he was still in primary school. He lived not very far away from where I had my house in Caprile and he frequently came up and stayed a little. But he was also quite without significance, *ja*, only an acquaintance. And then I had another acquaintance; a certain Desiderio, a businessman from Capri . . . a bear of a man, gay and happy, who also knew my friend Frieda Schutzl who lived in Anacapri. She was the housekeeper of Clavel, the rich hunchback who danced with Don Domenico and who had a villa in Capri. She liked Desiderio, and I liked him also, it was a very comfy story. No jealousy. I also liked going down to the Marina Piccola with him, when the visits were over, before I went up to Anacapri.

When Giulietta was in Switzerland and I was left alone with Andrea, I would telephone up to him in

Anacapri in the evening after the visits and say: 'Make some porridge, make this, make that.' The whole of Capri knew about this, because the telephone is a public one in a *patisserie*. I had no longer a maid, and so I would telephone him up there: 'Now cook and get this or this ready.' And he would go to the phone, and he would also take messages for patients, and when someone rang—he was still only a boy—he would say: 'Now Mama is in the Marina Piccola, now she is in the Marina Grande, and if you want to catch her,' etc., and when I came home, he would tell me, this or that person had rung.

But because he was a boy, he would be down in front of the house, and play ball and romp with the boys, and run in to the telephone. But he did everything and was good at giving messages. He always did this, and that's why everyone liked him, and (you know how they love to gossip in Capri) wherever I telephoned from, they would then tell this to Edwin Cerio, and he then once made a whole list of what I had ordered Andrea to do, what Andrea was to cook for us to eat—he had written out a whole menu very beautifully, painted it, one could almost say, first oatmeal, then absurd names he made up as a joke like *Pollo Spiatore* (spy chicken), *Carne alla Zuffa Sanguinosa* (meat from the thick of the fight)—a whole menu with absurd wines at each course. He was a satirist. But you must have read his books.

In the meanwhile, it's true, there was just a little time left for Desiderio and the schoolmaster.

Then I met a Dutchman, he lived at the Punta Tragara in a very beautiful villa, and I had attended him together with a friend. This friend was Fred Brachet, a homosexual, and he had been very ill. He was not pleased with his Capri doctor because he didn't seem to improve, I think he had jaundice, and so this Dutchman whom I knew, said, 'Now call in the Dottoressa.' Brachet didn't want to because he was a homosexual, but then he did call me in and grew to like me quite a bit. It was no sexual relationship because he was, after all, in that other way. But he was nice and kind, and he recommended me around to his boy-friends, to all who were there, so I became quite a fashion, and they would then invite me to the various dinner parties they had there, and I would treat the boy-friends, and when one of them had something wrong with him I was of course called in, they were not at all ashamed, not at all, no. But the marvellous thing was, one of them would kiss the other one, and then he would come and kiss me, and then he would go back and kiss his other boy-friend. It was strange and so natural too. And the Dutchman, he was not one of those, he was a very serious man, a very refined man, well read, and he had women friends, quite a few of them. He went to some and a few came to him. It was a large house, where there was always someone; like a dovecote. I think with most of them he had platonic friendships, as he did with me. I almost believe it was as if he wanted to have women around him although he moved in homosexual circles, and although the young men came also, he also invited women . . . He had been Professor in Utrecht, he had had a chair in Utrecht. It was a beautiful friendship.

There was even one time, but that was much later after the war, when I arranged what you might call a little wedding. There was this Englishman whom I met at the house of an Austrian lady. She was the *petite amie* of a great man who made all the best jam which you

130

bought in all the shops—cherry, blackcurrant, everything. There was always jam in her house, but he gave
her much else beside. He was an honest man and he
looked after her even when he was dead. Always in her
house were homosexuals, dozens of homosexuals, and
cats, hundreds of cats. I exaggerate, yes, but a little
only. There I met this elderly Englishman and he had
fallen in love with an Anacaprese boy, he was crazy, he
didn't know what to do, he lived in a hotel, you see. So I
told him, 'I will make you a little wedding dinner in my
house,' and I did it very nicely with candles and a good
Anacapri wine, and then I left them to get on with it.
Once I wanted to be a nun, you remember. Well, I was
a little bit of a priest with that wedding. They were
happy with that dinner. Did I not do right?

Seeing Gigi Again

In what year are we now? '32, '33? Then Hitler was
in Germany. Now comes a good joke! There I lived in
Capri and I never read a paper, only the *Corriere dei
Piccoli*, and once when Ludovico came down to visit us
in the holidays, he was always talking about Hitler, and
so I said, 'Who is that as a matter of curiosity?' And he
says: 'What, you don't know *that*?' I had no idea what
was going on.

Of course about Mussolini I had some idea. Not at
first but afterwards, yes. I knew about him through
Tutino, because Tutino, when Mussolini did his *Marcia
su Roma*, happened to be in Naples, on duty. Why I no
longer know, but at any rate they were all called up in
those days.

In the year 1933, a family of rich landowners, von

Landen, from East Prussia, invited me to spend the holidays at their property in East Prussia, in Klein Guja. Whether I had met them in Capri, that I don't know, but I had met them as patients. They were interested in me and said it was about time I went away from Capri, I was too anaemic in Capri, and it was high time I had a change of air in the holidays, it would assuredly be good for me to go north. And so I went. At first I went via Innsbruck, and I invited my son Ludovico to Innsbruck, with his father, with Gigi, and we went together to Rinn which is above Innsbruck and spent a few weeks there.

It was funny to be with Gigi again and pleasant. Gigi no longer lived in Vienna, he lived with his mother in Basel, and had a liaison with a certain Baseler. Gigi had inherited a lot of money from his father and he opened some industrial concern in which this Baseler helped him, and Ludovico went to school there and lived with his father. Of course Gigi still painted and earned with his painting, but apart from that, he wanted to put the money to good use, and of course the whole lot was lost with speculations.

He was not as beautiful as when young, because he was fatter, but he was still a beautiful man, and he still grieved about me, as his mistresses told me. Zuzzi said this as well as the one in Basel. When he was a little bit full of wine in the evenings he would cry, and he would tell them how lovely it had been with me and he wanted me again, so in his cups there was still this love. He liked to drink, he already did as a young one in Positano with Don Domenico; *bottiglioni* came there, they didn't merely drink, they boozed five litres, put it away like nothing—five litres! But that was very good wine, a natural wine, there was none of this mixed stuff.

As for his women . . . on the whole he liked small, delicate ones, yes, Zuzzi was small, but that Czech, she was large, but then she was a model, and he always had his models whatever size they were.

So we stayed in Rinn, near Innsbruck, and it was still very lovely with Gigi and Ludovico, they had forgotten their passport, but that did not seem to matter so much in those days. Not like now, my God!

Ludovico at that time didn't talk about our not being together again, but thereafter he suffered a lot, and he had the longing to bring us together, the more so because Gigi would get these crying fits and actually wanted me, and so he saw it all from his side, and on the other hand he knew all about Tutino. He was, after all, eighteen! And Andrea—he was with me. I could not have left him all alone in Capri.

In East Prussia

So we left Gigi and went north and when we got to Munich, I wrote to those von Landens, that I wasn't alone with Andrea but that I was bringing also the son from Switzerland, if this was all right with them, but I didn't wait for a reply because we were already on the way. We travelled via Berlin and via Koenigsberg where Ludovico got tipsy for the first time in his life, in the Blutgericht—and yes, it was there too during the first war, I got tipsy when I was pregnant and now twenty years later, Ludovico went to the same place to which he had been before, in a manner of speaking, as a non-existent child, and he got tipsy too. He began to feel horribly sick, poor Ludovico, and I was cross with him, and he was so unhappy. And there was a tremendous muddle, because he had broken a basin or something, so that we had troubles with the people whose place it was. This was certainly the first time he got tiddly, the wine was definitely very strong.

And then we went on, because it is a long way away, it is almost at the lakes of Masuria, Klein Guja. They were highly placed, those Landens. They had around seventy horses, and heavens knows how many cows. They were real *Junkers*, very rich people.

They did not mind that Ludovico was with me. They only said: 'Why didn't you say this earlier?' On the other hand as a Prussian von Landen was fearfully punctual. In the morning, all had to be at breakfast, to the split second all went to bathe in the lake. It was a lovely lake, and there was shooting where they shot those poor birds, the wild duck, and whatever else there was. And it all ran according to a time-table, organised to the last second. A very strict gentleman, he was. He interested himself in politics of course, he was a real *Junker*. His wife and his daughters were there also. They were very well brought up, and it was all very strict. Little Andrea was put on a horse and was allowed to ride, and I still have the most lovely photos of him sitting on a horse. He was frequently thrown off, but that doesn't matter, does it?

Von Landen often took Ludovico on excursions, and once there was a huge lobster feast (those are the sweet-water lobsters), and there was always wine to drink, though not enough to get tipsy, oh no, and then there were the fruit soups, when one got home from the woods, delicious cool fruit soups . . .

134

We were there for the whole summer, and then we returned. Ludovico went back to Basel and Andrea and I to Anacapri.

Now we are coming nearer to the war and to all the terrible things ... That summer was beautiful and happy. Why does God make us pay so much to be a little happy?

An Urgent Call from Basel

We settled in. I had these many patients, and after some months of it, there came one morning, quite early, the telephone bell at the *patisserie*, and the operator said: 'Dottoressa, what is the matter? We have been trying all night to get hold of you, we have an urgent call for you from Basel. Your son is dangerously ill in the clinic, you must go at once.'

I managed to throw on something, the handbag with the passport and money I grabbed, the shoes I only put on in the bus, and I went down on to the Marina Grande, and crossed with the boat so that I could catch the early morning train to Basel. A horrible journey with the fear of death on me all the time. In Rome I telephoned again while I was changing trains and got the answer: 'Yes, yes, please come.' And so I arrived in Basel, and I found Ludovico in the clinic and spoke with Professor Henschen who said to me: 'Well, you must understand that this is a double perforation, the appendix and the other gut, with an inflammation of the peritoneum. We are trying to pull him through with a new method. With a duodenal probe. Through the nose, down into the duodenum. I have had one case, a solitary case. I think he had come from the Balkans, and it succeeded, but many other times I have known it to fail. The probe sucks the pus out of the intestine.'

It is a terrible thing to be a doctor and to understand all that doctors say—and even what they don't say. In those days there was no penicillin. On the third day my colleague, the Professor, said: 'We hope we'll pull him through. He is putting up a good resistance.' And then he wanted to know if he had been breastfed, and I said, 'Yes, nine months long.'

'Well, then we hope we'll pull him through.'

Then he regained consciousness, and after all it was all right that time. I was given some years of that one as though God rations things like a cruel father. 'Yes, one more helping you may have but no more.'

Ludovico remained in Basel of course, and I went back to Capri to Andrea. Then for the first time, I noticed, that which I had never noticed before, that there was an enormous difference in the air and the climate on the island. Although it was May, in Capri there was a much thinner and better air. Yes, it was like a rebirth. You see, it wasn't only that Ludovico was getting better, that he had pulled through, it was that of course as well, but it really was something in this Capri air, and I noticed it for the very first time. Afterwards I noticed it every time. In the following years I travelled up and down, and it didn't matter what time of year it was, when I got on the boat and went across to Capri, I had this feeling of being revitalised. It's exactly what the scientists say, an emanation we have in Capri from Monte Solaro. That is a revitalising emanation, radio-activity perhaps, because it is the only high elevation which lies in this part of the gulf on an island. All the other elevations are on the mainland over there. When

136

one comes newly and straight to Capri one notices it, as I now noticed it. Revitalising, rejuvenating, *joie de vivre*, working strength, all this in the first days. It doesn't last long, perhaps one or two days. Later you are used to it, but it is there all the time, and so it is things happen in Capri like nowhere else, funny things, curious things, and sad things.

The Black Princess

I had to go to the Marina Piccola, to the house of an Italian princess, whom we all called the Black Princess, the *Principessa Nera*. And it was for this reason: because of mourning her lover whom she had lost suddenly, she had everything in the house in black. The napkins were black, the sheets black, the pillow-cases black, everything was black. Also the table-cloth, it too was black. A curious vulgarity, like Sarah Bernhardt sleeping in her coffin. Only her skin was white. White like a clown, like snow. With black all round her eyes, and black mouth, black painted nails and toenails. She was between thirty and forty, or perhaps even older. Yes, and she became really old, for she was still in Capri when the war was over, and she remained the same, black as night. She was never seen until it was dark and then sometimes you would see her in Gemma's restaurant. Graham Greene told me he once had lunch with her and her lover—a new lover—on the beach at the Marina Piccola in front of her house and there was all the blazing sunshine and she was black, all black, and Graham didn't like his lunch because she had a lot of Pekineses who ran over the table and ate out of the dishes.

But this day was years earlier, before the war, and I was suddenly called late in the evening. I must go to the side of the Marina Piccola, right at the top, and I found there the lattice standing open. I rushed in and coming towards me was a man, bleeding from a cut face. There were cuts right down to his throat, bleeding profusely, and a woman unconscious on the bed, or sofa or whatever it was. So in the first instance I had to see what was up with her. There was a sort of smelling-salt which I gave her and felt her pulse, and it was there. I splashed her with cold water and all the things one does in a case like that. In the first moments, without anyone to help, I could not attend the man. He sat in front of a basin and the blood just ran and he tried to wipe it and to stop it. I told him: 'Hold it quiet. Do not dab.' He could not speak. When she regained consciousness and he succeeded in keeping back the blood from his wounds, then . . . the whole thing had been nothing but a fight; they had begun to quarrel and she grabbed his razor and inflicted the wounds, and he had to defend himself, and so doing the cuts went hither and yon, and when she saw what she had done, she fainted again. This time I tended his cuts and left the black and white maniac in her trance. The man was her lover—not the one who died of course. It had been an affair of jealousy, you see. He stayed at home for a week, so no one saw him, and pretended to have a bad cold, or a bad stomach, he pretended some such thing. She hid him because he was not supposed to be seen with her. As for the other, the one who died, he was a sort of lion in society, a drawing-room lion, who every day chased around with her.

The Compton Mackenzies

This may have been about the time when Compton Mackenzie, the English writer, lived with his wife on the Tragara in a lovely house, and his wife met a Russian in Capri. She went one night with the Russian whom she had met shortly before this, and whom she was very much in love with, and crossed over to Sorrento in a fishing-boat. In the morning Mackenzie alerted the whole of Tragara, everyone, everyone he alerted, the servants and everybody. Then it transpired she had gone in the fishing-boat, which they had hired from a fisherman, and she went off with the Russian, she went off for good. She must have been around thirty, a tall beautiful woman, a voluptuous one.

The Russian was a tenor. He was a big Russian, like they often are. Who knows better about Russians than I do?

After a lot of years had passed she came back. Mackenzie was long since living in Scotland, but she came back with the Russian. The villa had been sold, so she came to a hotel in Capri, and they called me, because she had a sudden heart-attack. High blood pressure, and walking uphill; she was near a stroke. I called one of the grey sisters immediately, and let blood. I did a thorough blood-letting with leeches on her temples, and I can still remember that during this process after big screams at the leeches, she kept asking for brandy and so finally in God's name I gave it to her. Because you know one shouldn't. Well, anyway, the black went from her eyes and forehead and the leeches were fat as hell, yes, yes . . .

The Russian was with her. So there they were both complaining about the leeches, oh my God. A long,

long time had passed since they went to Sorrento in the fishing-boat. They had become very sedate, and the Russian was most dignified . . . they were companions now, not lovers. Then they again left, and I lost them. At the end her eyesight was failing and I'm told she fell backwards down a whole flight of stairs to the basement. That was the end of poor her.

Axel Munthe

In Anacapri, of course, the most famous man was Axel Munthe, the lover of the Queen of Sweden. All the people hated him because he tried to stop them netting and killing the quails. He felt himself of great importance because he had written that famous book about San Michele and because of the Queen of Sweden. She had her house in Anacapri and he had his apartment in the palace at Stockholm, and the King of course was very content because he had his tennis and his young men.

Munthe was a very smooth man. Norman Douglas had an expression for him. He said he was a 'portentous fake'. Edwin Cerio, too; he thought him absurd. About this famous bird-sanctuary of Anacapri Cerio wrote that Munthe had truly created a Paradise—for hunters. Once before the first war I saw him and the Queen walking with Kaiser Wilhelm from Caprile, where the Queen had her house, down to Materita, to Munthe's tower. Wilhelm was in uniform and Munthe had a straw hat on his head and a light summer suit. He remained a pace behind them, and he looked very preoccupied. I have the impression he was smiling about the two in front of him, with satisfaction. Two royal people going to his tower.

No one who was important enough could escape Munthe. Even Greta Garbo. I saw her on the path down to Materita, in a summer dress, quite light, with a summer hat, as one wore then, with a little veil in front of her face. She was running down the path to Munthe's, so light she was, all I had was an impression, but what a beautiful impression.

I met Munthe first with the peasants. At Maldacena's, in the Piazza Boffe. A man was paralysed through a heavy stroke. I was called in as general practitioner, and Munthe came as consultant. And he said to me, 'I have heard so much about you, you do so much good for these good people, and you come to visit them,' (medically). And then he invited me to San Michele. He said: 'When you have time, come and lunch with me. But I have a very large sheepdog and you will be sure to be afraid of him. So you'll have to go to the peasants, the ones who look after everything. You'll have to go to them, because otherwise the dog will leap at you too much.' And so I said, 'Well I am not afraid of any dog,' and I went down round about lunch time, when he had invited me, and was let in, and the big dog immediately leapt up at me on to my shoulders, his head higher than mine, for I am small, and he was a large Alsatian. But he only leapt at me, and immediately was nice and I was not at all afraid. And I can still remember that Munthe said: 'Look, look at that; he seems to like her.' Such behaviour seemed to astonish him!

Then we had lunch. And they had warned me beforehand, 'You know, for lunch you won't get much, not in that house. You needn't think you will.' And so I had the lunch, and it was macaroni and vegetables. With it a glass of red wine. Finished. He discussed the various cases about which one had told him, and asked my opinion, it was more medical than private. And he was happy that I was on such good terms with his dog, because I rushed around with the dog all over the property and he laughed.

It is very lovely, San Michele, but he showed me nothing. About the collection I was only told by the peasants who ran his house, they showed me all that, but he himself, not. He only invited me to lunch and then we walked in the garden with the dog, Gorp. You find this name not strange? Gorp? And then I went to eat with him another time and he wanted to speak very privately with me, and he said he now knew me and I was to promise him something. His big worry was his last hours, when his life's end would come. When he was approaching his life's end, he would send for me and I should come and I was to stay with him, and when there was nothing more to be done, he said, 'You must promise me you will give me a morphia injection which will allow me to sleep quietly during my way across. You will promise me that.' He said, 'Please always remember this.' And I said, 'Good, yes. When life is leaving you.' Then he said, 'I know by my experience and because I now know you, as a doctor that you will do it, within the framework of our profession.' I had to promise him that.

During his absence he had a cataract operation, and when he returned, I came out of my house and met him, wearing one of those grey summer suits, walking with a straw hat on his head. He said, 'Ah, it's you, yes, you know that this is exactly how I imagined you would look!' Because before his operation he could only see me very dimly, he practically didn't see at all. It was what is called a black cataract. 'It's exactly how I imagined you would look. And tomorrow you must come to me; I brought you such a lovely book, it's called *Beautiful Switzerland*.' He wrote nicely in it for me, and I still have it today. And then I went frequently down to see him. And he gave me his main work *San Michele* with photos. There are only a few of this edition. The ordinary books in all languages are without photos. This one is beautifully illustrated and he wrote me a dedication in it.

The war came, and we had to go. I went to Switzerland from Berchtesgaden. I'll tell about this later, and in the second or third year of the war, Munthe travelled to Stockholm with his secretary, who was a boy of the peasant family who did for him. To Sweden they went and he died in the Royal Palace in Stockholm.

As for Munthe's famous book I only like the end, the dream sequence, the fantasy which is no longer reality. At first the book held my attention, but it is quite different from Capri as it is, the real Capri. It was a dream Capri, like clouds, not like those dangerous limestone crags which are Capri. But when Norman Douglas called him a 'portentous fake' he was not fair. Munthe was a solitary, an original. He could, under some circumstances, be very theatrical, there perhaps he faked, and then again he would become a simple person, modest, depressed, quiet, almost silent . . . Norman liked only knowledge—Munthe's world was a little chimerical, and Norman despised this. He felt only contempt for the 'afterlife' to which Munthe paid such great attention.

At that time there was not much talk about the Swedish Queen. Nobody bothered, it was a time when no one thought very much about these things. In fact, no one bothered with foreigners. The Caprese took them as they came, they were of another world, which the islanders didn't have much to do with. If they had money, that was what was important, but not to the *contadini.*

Count Fersen

At that time too on Capri there was the Count Fersen. In Compton Mackenzie's book *Vestal Fire* you will find him, and Roger Peyrefitte wrote a whole book about him called *The Exile of Capri.* In Mackenzie's novel he is called Count Marsac. His villa was that villa you can see on the edge of the cliff of Capri near the Villa Jovis, the Palace of Tiberius, and like the Palace it has a precipice which drops straight down. There in a green garden stands the house, quite in the wilderness, and the garden has become a jungle out there on the rock. And this Count Fersen—Fersen is a Swedish-French family, I think—had built this place and lived there with his general factotum who was also his boy-friend. A homosexual, yes. He had of course other servants, it was very luxurious. And Clavel, the Swiss hunchback, who now had a villa in Anacapri with his housekeeper Frieda, he would visit Fersen often and together they smoked opium in this oriental retreat which Fersen had had designed for the purpose. One day they would smoke in this villa and then again in a villa in Anacapri and the boy-friends came, and all sorts of other people. It was a closed circle, though a large one. Yet at other times Fersen would be very conventional in society.

So it went on, this exotic, rich and illusioned life until one fine day they found Fersen dead. The major-domo, his friend who was Italian, never really told the whole story, not even to the family who then came from France to his funeral. No one ever really discovered the full story. One morning, there he was, dead. The family, they were pretty distant relatives, asked no questions, they hushed it up, and the villa remained empty, slowly rotting away because nobody bothered about it, this beautiful but inaccessible retreat.

On a Sunday afternoon much later I once walked past and I climbed through a hedge and saw it all. Some of the furniture had disappeared, and some of it was still standing there and the garden trees had made a jungle; it was so sad. There was talk once of turning it into a *pensione*, but nothing came of that, so remote it is and too difficult to reach. You may walk if you are strong and not in a hurry, or ride up on a donkey. There is no road up there. Of all that oriental life nothing was left except a small tin of opium which Fersen gave me I don't know why—a joke, a whim. That tin many years later I gave to Graham Greene because he told me how he smoked opium in Indo-China, and one night in London with a friend he remembered it and they opened the tin and smoked Count Fersen's opium, thirty years after he had died, in Albany off Piccadilly. But they had no proper lamp and a lot of the opium dripped on the bed and made a great smell, but there were no police dogs sniffling around in those days. Graham told me it was beautiful opium. It had lost nothing in all those years after the Count had died.

Capri in those days was quite a centre for homo-sexuals of both sexes. Perhaps it was its reputation from the time of Tiberius and being an unreal sort of place of such beauty, and this was the time too when there came from Germany military high-ranking officers who would quarter themselves in a hotel. And there was the whole Krupp affair. Friedrich Alfred Krupp—the King of Guns Cerio called him. It was he who built that path down to the sea, to the Piccola Marina. A multi-millionaire, and yet he killed himself, poor man, be-cause of a scandal with a boy. They hounded him.

Later after the first great war Norman Douglas came back to Capri and lived there, and it was again like the old days, for there were his friends and the young boys to whom he gave sweets like Don Domenico—you can imagine for what—and all the Lesbians were there as well. But then the second war came, and those days never really returned again. All the rich bourgeois came from Rome in the summer and the day-trippers from Naples and the Americans wearing paper hats. It was not the same. It was a police island too. People were afraid. Even Norman. No, he was not afraid, but his friend Kenneth Macpherson in whose house he lived was afraid for him and told him he no longer could have those children to the house, but that is another story.

Norman was in danger because of his boys. Malaparte was expelled because he wrote something bad about the island in a newspaper, and once all the fishermen were sent over for trial in Naples, poor them, for living off the money of the American women who came alone to Capri for holidays carrying price lists—Giovanni

10,000 lire down to poor Enrico 1,000. There was one poor fisherman who loved, truly loved, an American girl with a monkey on her shoulder. She had no money and she made him pay for everything. She even asked me and Graham to have dinner in a fine restaurant and made the fisherman pay. But the police sent him across to Naples with the rest, and when he returned she was gone to Rome and he wept, poor man.

I will tell you one story to show how people were afraid in Capri just after the war. One night Graham Greene had a little party in Gemma's restaurant—there was I and Cavalcanti, the film director, and Aniello, the builder, and everyone had drunk too much except me. It was a little before the elections. (What elections they were! The Communists used the head of Garibaldi on their posters and all the nuns voted for them because they thought it was the head of St Joseph). Well, Graham, because he was a little drunk said, 'Here in Gemma's we will hold our own elections, and you, Cavalcanti, will be a candidate for the Communists because you have just come from Czechoslovakia and you, Aniello, will be for the Christian Democrats, and I will be for the Anarchists.' The *pizzeria* was full of people, not a table was empty, and Graham began to make a speech for the Anarchists and everyone left the *pizzeria* quickly, not finishing to eat, except one man who sat alone, and Aniello said, 'Be quiet, Graham, that is the Chief of Police.' So the fear was in Capri in those days. The fear went, but nothing was the same again.

But you must not think I spent all my time with famous people. This was not my real life. Each morning Andrea went to school at the Certosa and we both went on foot down to Capri by the Phoenician steps. I would open my surgery, and then at one o'clock I fetched Andrea and we went back up to Anacapri, climbing all the way—*Mamma mia*, what a climb that would be for me now—and I cooked some lunch for us both very quickly. Then, of course, immediately afterwards, down again for the afternoon surgery, and following that the visits in Capri and in Anacapri, where Andrea somehow must cook something for supper as I wasn't home at all till night. He knew how to cook. He liked to do it. Andrea ran the house, and I ran to do my visits. Although he was only round eleven or twelve. But he had mature ways as well as the wildness of boyhood . . . Ah, yes . . .

There are terrible things that happen with the poor. Capri is not only an island of pleasure. It is an island of much pain, especially in the winter when all the tourists are gone. I remember how late one night I was called to the Catena. The Catena is one of those streets which goes from below Monte Solaro up in front of San Michele, the home of Axel Munthe. Up there are four old farmhouses. And there I found in one of those farmhouses a sturdy, strong peasant lying on the bed with the baby half in, half out. She was in the middle of the birth and without help. If only someone had told me that it was a birth, but 'Hurry up and come!' is all they said. And when I arrived I found this woman and had to turn the child, it was very difficult. All instruments for birth were in my bag at home. One arm was already out, the other wouldn't go: in short, the baby was dead, but I could save the woman. The child had suffocated. It was much too large a baby, it was a breech birth, so you see it would have been a difficult birth in any case. And it was my first difficult birth on Capri. As a rule the women never even bother to fetch a midwife.

Many years later, after the war, I was called up again to the Catena. But this was a young girl who had not told anyone that she was pregnant, and now was the time of the birth. She lay in a shed, not even on a bed. The child was already out . . . I had to use a piece of string which lay there, in order to tie off the umbilical cord, and I found a pair of shears, and I gave her first aid. She had been slow about calling me. To say it was a birth—that would have been for her the end. Because they have terrible scenes with their parents, who would then make the boy marry the girl. So it happened this time. He married her. He was threatened . . . so he had to marry her. In the end everything was in the best order. Now they have a grocery store, and she had several other children . . . All things on Capri do not end so happily as that.

One evening they called me that I should come quickly to a hotel, yes, to a waitress. She was said to be ill with colic. Well, I arrived and by the bed I found a newborn child, dead.

I don't know to this day if she killed it or if it was a stillbirth. I only know the infant lay there, and that I helped her with the afterbirth, and that she begged me with tears in her eyes that no one in the hotel should know of her confinement, and this I managed to do. I took the child with me in my big bag and buried it underneath my orange tree. That's where it lies to this day, and no one has ever found out. She was so very young, and I thought only of her; she was a German to boot. And she was very plucky. Two days later she stood again in the dining-room and waited on people. In the meantime I had buried it and no one knew. Everyone thought she had had an intestinal colic.

I think I was right, to do this for her. Think of the police and the investigations and the prison in Naples. It was bad enough for her to have the child, no?

As a doctor, I should have declared it. But I was at peace with God, and had no feeling of guilt. On top of it all, burying the little body was extremely difficult, for it was summer and the earth was hard like rock. Me with a big spade. People can't see into my garden because of the high wall, but how hard it was. When it was done I was weak and shaking as a jelly. As soon as the season was over she paid me what she could, what she had earned honestly . . . That she gave me and from Germany after the war she once sent me a postcard.

In Capri one must not tell everything to the authorities. One must be quiet also and secret. Even when Norman Douglas died I did not tell . . . but that I must describe later. Now I am in my little garden with my orange tree, with the big spade. Often there later I had to bury cats. When I had my big boxer, when a cat came into the garden, he would toss it in the air and kill it. He was not popular in the village. People were afraid of him and if they had known what happened to their cats they would have gone to the *carabinieri*, but he was right, the cats had no business in my garden, and so I would bury them where I buried the child. Once in winter the ground was too hard, and a cat when it dies, it is heavy like Hell. Graham and I took one handle of my bag each and we walked out of Caprile to find somewhere to dump the body and Graham complained all the time that the cat was too heavy and every time we stopped to throw away the body there were the lights of a car coming down the road. Never had there been so many cars at night on that road.

I will tell you another story. It was on a Sunday, and I was down in Mesola. Mesola you find when you go towards the lighthouse, down from Anacapri, and then you turn right to the sea, before you get to the Axel Munthe tower, and it is lovely down there. An Englishwoman or an American had bought this Mesola, and I was invited there. And quite by chance, Ludovico, my son, was there for the holidays. He was already at university. Well, we were down there and on this Sunday we came home quite happily when suddenly—telephone—I was to run fast, fast to the Hotel Eden Paradiso. And there I found a young German girl, in the bathtub in a pool of blood, who begged me to do what I could; I should help her as she was bleeding to death. And it was a tear in the vagina. The penis had been too big and she was torn, a heavily bleeding tear. A very deep wound. In such a case one has to stitch it. And in that moment, I had nothing with me. I could only use gauze, which I had quickly fetched from the chemist's, and I made a tampon. I made a big tampon and at the same time telephoned a colleague of mine, because it was on a Sunday and he was there from the hospital in Naples, and he came up and together he and I sewed her up.

These cases are not so rare as you think. During the war, a much worse case occurred in Switzerland, in

Lucerne. It was a Negro and a Swiss girl, and it was like this: they had got stuck inside each other. It needed two or three doctors to help to undo them. Such dreadful injuries. And the Negro, he was like a wild animal . . . quite terrible. Well, with the German girl, I found her alone, and with the aid of my colleague was able to do a good job of work. That was a thing which was only frightful for the moment. She healed very well and came to my surgery to visit me, but I never found out who the man concerned was.

Yes, for a doctor it was certainly an island of pain and not only for the poor. There was the poor American woman who had a lot of money and lived in a house below the Due Golfi on the way to Marina Piccola. She wanted to make a sort of artistic salon and she entertained many people. There was Pucci, the dress designer (he used to put on a different shirt between every course). She even managed once to catch Graham—it was very difficult to refuse her invitations because she had lunches so many days in the week and in Capri, except for a doctor, it is difficult to say, 'No, on Monday I am engaged, on Tuesday too, and Wednesday is not convenient.' She made acquaintances, but she did not make friends, and one day she took a lot of sleeping pills and to make sure she cut her veins open over the bidet. When she was found dead people came in and stole everything from the house, even her clothes. I do not blame them too much, they were poor, and she had no more use for anything. But the funeral—that was ignoble. Of all her friends only the Dutchman, Tony Paanaker, went to the funeral—perhaps it was out of season, I cannot remember, but what I do remember is how the undertakers, before they put the coffin in the ground, unscrewed all the brass handles and put them in their pockets.

That is sad, but it is also funny and perhaps that is the worst. There was Lady Green who was put in prison in Naples. That cannot be a good experience, but how can one not laugh a little?

Before the war Lady Green had a lover who was a Spanish bull-fighter and she tried to persuade Mussolini to allow bull-fighting in Italy. I don't know what happened to the bull-fighter. After the war Lady Green, who was an old lady then, lived alone in her house with a young manservant who was very susceptible. If she had a male guest, her valet would write little notes and poems and put them on the tray with the *petit déjeuner*, telling of his love, and that was not always appreciated.

Lady Green played the guitar and she was a kleptomaniac. One day she stole a cheque book from one of her guests and she sent her manservant across to Naples next day to cash a cheque which she had forged, but he was arrested on the boat, and Lady Green and he were sent to prison in Naples. I think her husband in England came and helped her out, but before that Graham went with a friend to spend a night in Sorrento, and the porter of the hotel said to his friend in a whisper, 'I am so glad to see that they have let you out of prison, Lady Green.' I think Graham was embarrassed a little, but she—no!

You see how it always is—in Italy we prefer someone who has been in prison. They are real people. Who would be friends with a *carabiniere*? Though sometimes you have to pity them too. One there was in Caprile who loved a girl in the house on the other side of the lane where I lived—he wanted very much to marry her, but she didn't want to marry him, and one night there was a boum! boum! and I ran down the lane. He had shot her and then he had shot himself. So even a *carabiniere* can have a heart.

The Co-respondent

Tony Paanaker—he was a curious one living alone with his Anacapri housekeeper and a pack of dachshunds in the huge white house he built and never finished because he ran out of money. They say he manufactured shoes when he was young and he became famous in England when an English lord divorced a young dancer who was his wife. She was called June and at first there were nineteen co-respondents for the lord to choose from and he chose the young foreigner Paanaker. Tony was very proud of that when he was an old man living in Anacapri in that villain of a house which was all wrong in the village. He liked women of an age and he would invite them alone for lunch and give them baked beans and Spanish fly. He had a bath with glass sides and he would lie in it naked and ask them to do things to him. Poor Tony! It cannot have been like that with the young dancer. He drank too like Hell. He was not a happy man, but Graham said his dry Martinis in a great glass jug were very good, though Tony always drank whisky.

One day when I was there and Graham and Norman's friend, Kenneth Macpherson, and Islay Lyons, we wanted to go home, but Tony we could not find. It was a wet day and Graham was looking for his coat and he opened a door in the hall and there in a little room sat five men in a row all dressed up in black as if they were in church. Later we knew who they were. They were the mortgagers.

That was a fine business Tony did. Everyone said, 'He cannot live long. He is drinking himself to death.' He was cardiac too and he had a blood pressure which ran up like a monkey on a stick. So these men agreed to pay Tony enough to live in the house and keep his garden clean and have cases of whisky and gin and when he died they would have the great white house and the glass bath. But then the years passed—more than ten I think—and Tony was still alive. The Anacaprese woman looked after him and cooked his food. No chance there of making him hurry a little towards death. She watched him like a hawk and no longer could he invite middle-aged ladies to eat baked beans. The mortgagers had spent more money than they could afford and so they had to find another generation of mortgagers and still Tony drank and drank and stayed alive.

Where is he now? He is dead like so many, like Compton Mackenzie and Kenneth Macpherson and Cecil Gray, like the murderer of Anacapri and poor Baron von Schacht, but it took more than twenty years of the mortgagers' money to kill that one. I am sad when I think of Tony, that hard man with his bad ways and no heart, but I am glad for him and I laugh like Hell when I think of the mortgagers.

The Anacapri Murderer

The murderer was the Anacapri barber. He had slept with a German girl on Monte Solaro, and as a result he strangled his wife, and threw her down the cistern in his garden. He got fifteen years' imprisonment, and did twelve of that, and then he returned to Anacapri and married again.

This murderer was a friend of Graham Greene's. Graham always had his hair cut by him because the barber would send out for a glass of wine to make him patient while he snipped. One night Graham gave a party at the restaurant in the piazza of Caprile for his friends. There was I and there was his friend Catherine and the Russian priest Father Ivan and Aniello, the builder, and Baron von Schacht and the murderer. He was not used to whisky and he had drunk too much at Graham's house and he complained that there was not enough food to eat. And then he pulled Catherine's hair and he caressed Baron von Schacht under the table with his murderer's hands. But this was too much. After that we danced on the piazzetta in a ring. Then Graham swung me round and round and to punish him I gave a great smack, but it was to Baron von Schacht it arrived. This poor one, what a night for him! Yes, I smacked the Baron hard and he had done nothing. I remember he cried out angrily: '*Das ist durchaus beschimpfend*! That is absolutely insulting! *Aber warum*?' I was laughing too much and he had then a very poor opinion of the Dottoressa. I apologised and explained how giddy Graham had made me, and then he too laughed and we danced. Oh, very stately. I came as high as the Baron's stomach which was not any more slender. That was a night!

Baron von Schacht

The Baron lived in Caprile on the way to the Migliera above a restaurant. He had come to live in Capri after the Kaiser's war, leaving his wife behind in Germany. When the Americans came to Capri in the second war they wanted to arrest him although he was an old man, but he was protected by the mayor. He had very little money and he was always hungry from the smell of cooking from the restaurant under his windows. Many people invited him to meals, and in gratitude he collected wild orchids on Monte Solaro which he brought as gifts to those who had been kind. If Graham was on Capri, always on his birthday in October would come very early a little boy with a great platter of little white flowers. You could say that after food little boys were the Baron's great pleasure as they were with Norman. He was a tall Prussian with big blue eyes and a shaven head, and he had been an officer in the Uhlans. In the little hall of his apartment was a photograph of his troop with the Kaiser on a white horse inspecting them, and he would give a big sigh and say, 'It was all so peaceful.' In a big wardrobe he kept his uniform, his helmet, his cuirass, his white gloves, and on the Kaiser's birthday he stayed alone and he dressed again in his uniform and sat there quiet and gleaming and hungry above the restaurant. Graham used a little of the Baron in his character of Hasselbacher in a book he wrote called *Our Man in Havana*.

After the war the Baron got a pension from Adenauer —not very much, but it killed him because then he wanted to return the hospitality of all those who had given him meals in the bad days. So he drank and ate too much—and perhaps too many of the other things he liked, now that he could give little presents to the boys. One day he drank a good deal and he went bathing at the Bagni di Tiberio and then walked up all the steep steps to Anacapri, and when he got to his room he had a stroke and he died immediately.

Next day there was a funeral and Graham had a great argument with the *carabinieri*, for Graham wanted to put the Baron's helmet and his gloves on the coffin for the procession, so that he would have a soldier's burial, but the *carabinieri* said it was the law that the apartment must be all sealed up with everything inside till the wife came from Germany and they said that thieves might steal the helmet. In the end Graham persuaded them that he would be responsible, and the coffin with the helmet on top went in procession down the street under the windows of the Eden Paradiso hotel. There the ex-King Farouk of Egypt in his exile had taken the whole top floor, and Graham said, 'Now he is looking down on us and seeing the funeral pass and what is he thinking? He will have to think about death instead of boiled eggs.' It was said that he would eat a dozen boiled eggs at a meal.

But what a thing is this memory. Here I am speaking already of the years after Hitler's war, but before all this happened I had lost Capri I thought it might be for ever.

An Exile from Capri

In 1937 I went to Germany in the summer. The Landens had been in Capri and they had found me seriously ill, with sweatgland abscesses of both armpits, completely exhausted. My colleagues helped me, they lanced me here, and then they lanced me there to drain the main sources of the suppuration, and the von Landen's found me in a heavily anaemic and pitiful condition, so they took me with them to East Prussia, because they said that I would recuperate with the good cows' milk and everything they had up there, as well as the northern climate. And so it was. At the end I had a very large abscess here on the hip, but with the good milk, it soon stopped.

I went with Andrea. He rode horses like a cowboy, very free and upright. On horses he was at home; he loved them as he loved all good things, only more. He loved all animals and landscapes and I must tell you something. At times I had this strange feeling which I tried to put from me, that I could not see him as old *ever*! He would stay not long on earth. Such radiant people never continue. He had a smile, I used to think, like June coming suddenly upon a dull November. And his body was good-looking. He seemed charmed. He was strange. A sort of Eros.

One of my patients was a certain Countess Waldersee. She was a descendant of the famous Waldersees. In gratitude for the treatment, although they always paid me, and also because they were interested in me, they invited us to their lovely house in Berchtesgaden.

Hitler was also in Berchtesgaden. He had that large house on top there, and to her home, to that lovely villa, came his Hitler Youths. Most schools had Hitler Youths, and first one class would come and then another, and she would put them up in the holiday-camp which she had next to her beautiful property. She let me come there with Andrea, who was given a lovely pair of *lederhosen* of which he was extremely proud, but she didn't want me to come into her house. Because, although I never actually said so, she noticed I was against this Hitler thing. I am not a discreet one and my disgust was evident. I found the ideology ridiculous, but more than that, disgusting, a poison. I didn't really know much about it, just its manifestations. This *Heil Hitler* and all that seemed to me to be tyrannical, infantile, terrible. This salute, this slavishness: all so drilled and unreal, like marionettes in a nightmare. Even today I am angry, when I remember it. My friends were as though they had been anaesthetised. They were so damped down, so crushed. They all said it, *Heil Hitler*, but I never saw any enthusiasm.

So there I was in Berchtesgaden, she had invited me, but she didn't want me in her home, so she put me into a modern chalet higher still up the mountainside. I was a clandestine one, in disgrace, though she was cordial when we met. Once or twice I saw Hitler when he went to the Koenigssee, from Berchtesgaden. Only for a moment as he went by. Solemn. Worried. Mad eyes. And lots of cars, a terrible thing in the lovely peaceful landscape.

So just before the outbreak of war, I was at this chalet of the Countess Waldersee above Berchtesgaden. She telephoned up to me, to tell me it would be better if Andrea and I were to come down. So we came down and I said, 'Well now, we must go directly to Switzerland.' What else could I do? So we went to Switzerland. First from Berchtesgaden to Lake Constance, and it was in Lindau on Lake Constance that I heard Hitler's speech at the outbreak of war. This was the speech where he started with: 'Our troops have marched into Poland,'—a tragic moment. Andrea ran on to the wrong boat. Foolish Andrea, even this delighted him, he laughed like a crazy one. I had to order him back. And then we went across to Switzerland.

When we arrived in Switzerland, my husband was dressed up as a home guard and my son too was in uniform ready to go to the army. There they stood and awaited us; 'It's good you came, and now you'll stay here.' Giulietta was through her studies at the horticultural school and she had a job as a gardener in Grundelwald.

Now it was a question of what to do. Not back to Italy and Hitler's friend, Mussolini. In Capri one had not noticed him, but here they spoke of how he would come into the war. Countess Waldersee had very much wished me to work in the hospital in Reichenhall, but Ludovico said, 'No, you won't leave Switzerland now. Be happy that we are all together. I am sure you will find something!' So I registered and was immediately given a long list of doctors looking for locums, because they had been ordered to do frontier duty. So then I did a locum; the first was with Doctor Gering from Biningen which is a suburb of Basel. He said, 'Well, you will be less worried, bring the boy, you can both of you be with me.' There were the usual duties of a locum. That is: in the morning I had to take the surgery, and in the afternoon all the visits, and Andrea was put into a secondary school first as a day-boy, but later when I left Doctor Gering's and went to various towns, he moved into the school as a boarder.

I represented Doctor Gering, which was quite something because I had to drive a car, and as you know, in Capri, I had only *seen* cars! For God's sake, to drive one of these things . . .

There was a painter, a young man who could drive

cars. He was someone who couldn't do his service, though he looked fit enough. Doctor Gering found him for me: I had to learn to drive as quickly as possible and had to take my driving test in two weeks. He came the next morning and said, 'Let's go and sit in the car,' so I got into the car, and he showed me how one had to do this. I could drive forward, that was easy, but to reverse, no. It was like Hell, this reverse. I could stop and I could go, but always I forgot all about this going back nonsense, and sometimes before I could park the car I must go a long way and then walk back. This reverse is an abominable affair. I never mastered it. Forward I could do it, but *Mamma mia*! this backside I cannot see.

Oh, I had accidents, of course. Once in Efretikon when I was beginning to go up a hill, a sledge with three boys got right under the car. Nothing happened to them. But to me there happened a lot. It was a frightful thing, my fear. I was not at fault, because they came charging down right under my car, so I stopped because I was going uphill. The children yelled. They were schoolboys with a little one as well. It was not serious, it was an uncomfortable thing. And then I had an accident which could have cost me my life. It was near Schaffhausen. I was coming back from visiting a patient. And on the main road, on the icy road I began to skid, and the whole car fell down a slope, head down and bottom uppermost. And the steering-wheel had me so firmly in its grip that I tipped the car the right way up and I was not badly hurt. Bruises, nothing else. But as for Doctor Gering's car, the steering was gone and the wheels too. The car had pretty far-reaching damages, yes, and the doctor had to pay. I had a police summons, although I had hurt no one. But then the bad thing was the doctor was not at home, but his bad witch of a wife, instead of understanding that a person who had had such a car accident needed a moment's peace, *not on your life*! The accident happened at noon, and there was the surgery in the afternoon, and in the evening, I had to go in another car to do the visits. That was too much, after such a shock I was quite befuddled.

That witch-woman had no insight. The Swiss women were impossible. They were all impossible. Cruel, heartless, one worse than the next, and so they still are.

So the years of the war went by. My colleagues were very nice to me and very satisfied, and I was asked to do the same locums over and over again. As soon as one was finished, another began. In my free time I went to see my son in the Tessin, and that was all. No private life at all. I was very good all those years. Like a saint I was. Driving and dispensing and visits and consultations. Eight to ten weeks I would spend as a locum for one doctor, and then there would be another. Always having to get used to a new car. One was a Ford, another a Mercedes, the third I forget. I tell you the kinds of cars that I was driving then don't exist any more. Never could the Dottoressa get used to those damned cars.

Gigi, my husband, I saw from time to time. When I came to Basel I would visit him. He got married at that time to a farmer's daughter. I was working at Doctor Staubli's in Emmenbruecke, and I had to ask for time off, in order to go to the wedding in Basel. To be present when your man remarries is quite a benevolent and condescending feeling. Like presiding at a charity-sale. And the girl she was nice and not put out at all by me, because I had been coming to the house often when

I was between locums. This marriage was the right thing for him because he had been too alone. She was a simple country girl. At this time he had grown big and fat. Someone had to tie his shoelaces. The beautiful Gigi! In his old age he still remained a handsome man. A big fat bear of a man. How shall I put it? Not a pale spongy man. His complexion was good. He was a colossus of a man.

Andrea came to the wedding too. He liked celebrations. Even nothing at all he would celebrate. We were all there. Gigi's children, my Andrea, some of his mistresses. Perhaps it seems a little funny. Always with me it is so. Ridiculous things and then bad things. His Leiner, the one who had helped him with his business, she was also present. Her he hadn't been able to have in the house because his grandmother was still alive, but she came to lunch and supper and so on and so forth. Leiner was my first successor, and only after that came Mugg—I find it not at all a romantic name.

These were all solemnly assembled. A peculiar *galère*, is it not? You see how behind the conventional life is hidden all this unrespectable débris. It is more sanitary, I think, to walk free as I did, for I did not have this fear to be found out. There is no impediment or need to mind narrow opinions. I tell you, to live as I have lived is wild, yes, but how could I wish it otherwise?

But this freedom, so precious to me, I risked to lose it all. I wanted so much to see Italy again. The Germans were still there. Applications seemed to take forever and there was no security in the whole thing, you understand. But in any case I applied. It was at the time when the Nazis were still in Rome. I had to get an attestation that I was of pure Aryan descent. For that rubbish, all was done in Vienna and through Germany, and I had to provide my whole family tree, the names and stations of all known predecessors. Well, thank God, I finally got this Aryan passport, and with this passport I could go to Rome. But only to Rome. Not to Capri.

So between two locums I went to Rome. Alone. Andrea remained behind. In Rome I wrote to my maid Virginiella in Capri that she should come to Rome. And she came and brought me what I needed. Certain papers, and all the things I wanted for the taxes. All those things she brought me to Rome and I was able to arrange things quite well, but that was not enough—I had this enormous wish inside me and I had this idea I might never see my house in Caprile again . . . I was always a pessimist all my life and it wasn't enough that Virginiella should come to Rome and bring me all the news. I had to see that island again myself, not just have news like stale fish.

In Rome I met an American woman, and this American had a severe tonsilitis and called me in. So I went to her and on her bedside table there was her passport. And suddenly I was struck by an idea. I looked into her passport because of the photo and I thought to myself, now, you will ask her for her passport and you will try to see if you can get down there with that passport. You can go to Capri. For an American it was possible because their country had not yet come into the war. So I took this passport, and she had such bad tonsilitis that she couldn't open her mouth, and my Swiss passport I left with the sisters in Rome, who had put me up. It was a big party I travelled with to Naples. I have no idea who they were. They were going on an excursion, you see. It was towards evening in summer when we had to get on the boat to Capri. And I had a scarf, a large head-scarf, and no one at the harbour recognised me. Because the danger was, and this I knew, that anyone in authority might have spotted me. I was well-known and I must not be recognised. They were friendly, oh yes, but they would have said immediately: the Dottoressa is here, she has returned, and then would have come the ones from the *Questura*, the *carabinieri*. The Dottoressa who had to leave because of the war. There wasn't a single Swiss there. No one is allowed to come. How come she is here?

Well, I got through, and when we arrived at the Marina Grande, I went straight to a waiting-room by the *funicolare*. It was already nearly dark, but I read a newspaper until night had quite fallen, and in the night I crept up the paths to Anacapri and to my house. I couldn't get in. I didn't dare, although I had the keys with me. All the same I saw my house, my Casa Andrea. It was such a happiness, but then after came the sad feelings. This terrible war and how it had fallen like a plague. Here at my house was peace as it had always been and all else was fear and death. So peaceful it was, this summer night. But I could not stay there. Each stone of every house on Capri was an eye watching. Of this you may be certain. The keys that would let me in were hot in my hand and I knew I could not use them. So, like a tourist, I walked on looking at everything. But it got late to be a tourist, and anyhow at this time a tourist was a bit peculiar, nearly all were away with the war, and the next time I passed my house I went straight by. It is easy to hide on Capri, so I hid, and the first boat for Naples it left early in the morning, stopping at Termini and Massa Lubrense and Sorrento and Vicovaro on the way. In the morning it was difficult. Because everyone came to the harbour, everyone I knew, but I succeeded because I was muffled up. I had this headscarf round my head. And I don't think that people could have thought of my being there. Not one of them recognised me. On the boat I pretended to sleep with my headscarf over most of my face. I saw people I knew but I avoided them in my corner seat.

That same day, I went back to Rome and returned to the ill lady, who was feeling better from her tonsilitis. She was happy when I gave her back her passport. I bought myself a fur coat. It was summer and all fur coats were much cheaper, and then with my Aryan passport, like a good girl, I returned to Switzerland and took up the next locum. I really had been very frightened, and when I told my children in Switzerland, they nearly beat me. 'Why, why do you do such things?' Everything had been fine with my house. It was closed for seven years, but when I came back after the war everything was as I had left it. Not even as much dust as there is now when one goes away. That I could not tell from the street, but I had seen my house—that was the great thing.

What an adventure it was—the lady in Rome and the false passport. There was also another little adventure with a German whom I met on the beach near Ostia. This the Germans allowed, that one should go to Ostia, it is so near to Rome. He was a nice German. I think he was an official at the consulate, and it seems to me that when I left for Capri, he came too as far as Naples. I don't remember exactly . . . That is the trouble. Gone is my good memory. I tell you that this old age is Hell! It was only a very small flirtation, but better than nothing. You see, I had become completely lightheaded in Rome. I had come from serious Switzerland, from all those locums and from this staid life in Switzerland. I came to Rome and in a matter of a few days I was completely changed. I bought on the black market. From America the Romans had packages, and some of the people sold these. So I bought myself some clothes, dirt cheap. As good as for nothing. And I went to the various restaurants. It was a much more lighthearted kind of life, and that's why I dared to travel down to Capri. I didn't consider the consequences, although there was such a to-do to get a permit which one had constantly to show. In the first days I had all the time to report to the Roman police in order to show that I was there.

After the war, I told people in Capri about my visit, but they did not believe me. Then they had to believe me, because I told them things I had seen to which they had to agree, and say: 'Yes, yes, she is right.'

'You are fine ones, you didn't recognise me!'

No one, thank God, no one did I meet when I slunk up there, not one of my intimate friends or enemies. It was all empty. In those days I could run, and I hastened up by the ancient steps, not by the road. Yes, up and then down again, without having anything, for I couldn't show myself in any of the cafés. All that night was without food or drink. And I couldn't show any light either . . . It was all a rashness. Because of the different air. I was like that in Rome too. People were less moral . . . They sat near the church of Santa Maria Maggiore on the church steps, and made love in all kinds of ways. Which one doesn't usually do in the street, no? The steps there are very wide, all the way round, and especially at night this was very convenient, and no policeman turned up. Yes, it was an immoral time, you could not see such things in Switzerland, my God no!

PART

4

Anacapri Again

How glad I was to leave Switzerland when the war was over. I succeeded in getting seats for myself and Andrea my son, with my dog called Tucci and three suitcases, on the second train that left Switzerland to Rome, and which took I think forty-eight hours. Tucci was a black cocker spaniel. I got him during the time of the locums.

The train came from the north, from Rotterdam and it travelled for ever ... Everywhere, everywhere, it stopped for ages. With three suitcases, we had packed everything so that we had enough provisions. We had heard that in Capri, where the American soldiers went to convalesce and rest, provisions were bad and scarce. I was told that it would be a good thing if we were to bring high-quality food and tins and such things. I heard it from Cerio, but in a roundabout way, through an Italian girl who had once been my maid, who could neither read nor write, so she wrote through a friend.

It was May 1946, when we at last arrived in Rome. We went to the German sisters until we could get a connection to Naples. They had a big bus for the first time, which went Rome–Naples, and that is what we took. From early morning a good half-day ... whereas now you can do it in three hours. We arrived in Naples, thank God, before the boat was due to leave, so we got on the ship—not one of those lovely passenger-boats they now have, it was one of those ones they had taken out of service during the war—and in that we went across and had to arrive in Capri before the twilight, before night fell ... There were no lights, no, no, no.

173

And from Naples I succeeded in ringing Cerio in Capri, and so he was at the Marina Grande with his car. He fetched us and took us to the Palazzo to sleep.

It was very good to see Cerio again. So many years had passed. It had been a great friendship. He was a nice man, impressive and so amusing. He would tease me, and I teased him and there was a little . . . well, there was a little sex with it, just light comedy. You understand for me it was . . . well, there had been with him an accident with a boat, and that had left him with no great thing—only a little thing had he got, and anyway with such an old one I didn't want to make love, he was ten years older than me and I had always had younger ones. But it was amusing all the same, we had fun together, and just this little spoonful of love. When I used to have dinner with him in the Rosaio in Anacapri, he would send his daughter Laetitia to have dinner in Capri, and after the war when I came back it went on in the same fashion a little. But now we were quite old, both of us.

Well, here I was back in Capri. On the first day I slept in the Palazzo, with Andrea and the dog, and on the next morning I drove up to Anacapri and opened up my house. It had been closed for seven years and no one had been inside it, no one had opened it up, no one had had a key. There was dust, yes, quite a bit, but compared with what I had imagined a house would look like . . . The wood was still good, but the paint was peeling and the mosquito nets were rotten, and, yes, the cistern had some things wrong with it . . . but on the whole . . . The lovely thing was the garden. The big climbing roses, which I had planted before the war, they were there, all by themselves. The Christmas trees, on the other hand, which I had planted in the last six years I had spent in the house before the war, these were all gone. Someone had stolen them, someone had got in. But the roses, they had collected them from the entire neighbourhood for every function, but they were only cut, and as it was in this month of May there was a lovely rose garden, and also the orange trees and lemon trees, all beautiful, yes.

My son and I we were very happy. Andrea had just done his Matura, so he was nineteen. And yet in a way, how can I say this? he seemed to be nineteen for eternity. Our relationship was the best possible one. The most lovely one. He loved only me. He felt nothing for Tutino. And this love, there was so much of it, it was so rich, and all people, all nature, he loved. Only Tutino he could not love. There was enmity there. You see, during the war Tutino had married a very young girl, and Andrea said that he did it so stealthily. Instead of writing about it with plain facts, it was done in a roundabout fashion. I only discovered it like that.

Tutino—I must admit—often had his doubts about whether he was really Andrea's father. He thought that perhaps Venacolocci in Pisa, the colleague who helped me with the medical finals . . . and Loggi yes, of whom he was also jealous. He knew nothing of the Air Force officer, and with that one, the colleague I had once in Capri, the snake, there had been nothing anyway. But he was jealous just in case . . .

Who *was* Andrea's father? Tutino, that I feel sure, and yet there was a mystery. My children always said, going by the resemblance which Andrea had, he must have been Tutino's son. The child had Tutino's mouth and yet other parts of the face were like Gigi's. Andrea

175

himself was a mysterious boy. His character was quite different from my other children. He was a real Italian. On the one hand, very gay, and on the other exactly the opposite. A combination of a very happy person, who then without warning was very far away like a single bird on top of a tree. Yes, a bird of passage. Not the weightiness of the German, but the lighter blood of the Italian. He had a tendency to melancholy, and to being sad. I had that also as a young girl. It was always so: blissfully happy one moment and sad like death the next. Yes, it was like that the whole of my life. Once up, and then again sad.

Andrea now could speak German. At first during the war when we came to Basel he couldn't speak a word of German, and in the Gymnasium he had to go into a class below his standard, because in Latin and other subjects he was good, but in German he was not good. But after six months the German teacher scolded the others, saying: 'Here is this boy from Italy, and now he writes me better essays, better compositions than you, you should be ashamed.' Yes, he was very gifted.

All my children were very fond of one another. Only with Ludovico and Giulietta there was a certain inner jealousy because they could feel I was fondest of Andrea. They teased me with this. 'Of course what Andrea does is always right with you.' And Gigi also loved Andrea, that was the best thing. He liked Andrea so much you would have thought he was his son. If I had not known that he wasn't really his son, I would even have thought it myself . . .

So there we were in Capri again, and naturally I must start planning. In the Palazzo Cerio, Cerio put two or three rooms at my disposal. We put the surgery furniture, the instruments, etc. on a small donkey, and brought it down from Anacapri. I began to practise medicine again and I was busy straight away, and in the morning Andrea quickly went down to the sea to bathe, and then quickly up again in order to make something for me to eat, so that I could eat without waiting. It was almost like the old days.

The Death of Andrea

On the 1st of August, it was a Sunday, we went down to the lighthouse. We ran down. There was beautiful sunshine, a superb storm had passed and cleared the air, and we arrived at the lighthouse where you may bathe. The sea had very high waves, terribly high waves. I said, 'Look at that, we won't be able to bathe.' And Andrea said, 'On this side, from this rock, it'll be possible.' And while I sat there, he put on his bathing shorts and stood up in the wind and jumped from the rock into the sea.

I looked at this sea as it came like explosions against the rocks, and I saw how low it sank and pulled and pulled, and then how it came forward pushing and pushing, breaking itself like big glass windows against the sharp limestone rock, sharp as razor edges; and I feared that this strong water would pick up Andrea and smash him upon those blades. This was my one fear even though he was a strong swimmer.

And then the men from the lighthouse feared quite the opposite, that he would be carried out to sea, for they ran out with a long rope so that he could hang on to it and so come back with the breakers. And (how may I explain this?) I did not really fear. Perhaps because

Andrea was powerful and athletic and swift and had sharp eyes and could judge when there were good opportunities. Also it was so beautiful a scene that it excited me.

But later I reflected that surely it was at this time that the real fear, the other fear which would have a real reason, entered me, although at first I did not recognise it, for it was greatly tempting for me to be out too in that water, to be living like something in the imagination of Homer. You understand? No, no, not a siren. No siren is the Dottoressa.

His teeth were very white and they were flashing, which meant that he was laughing and perhaps calling as well, but you could hear only the big noise of the sea and the wind. And there came also some of the Capri gulls which are called laughing gulls, for they make this loud sound like a cruel laughing, and they live, all of them, on the Faraglione Rocks near the Marina Piccola and come out and laugh whenever there are storms.

And the men from the lighthouse, they were my friends, they said, 'This son of yours, what a *pazzerello*!' What a mad one! And I said, 'Yes, but I want to go in too.' And one of them said, yes, we all know *you're* crazy, and I agreed they were right, and we all said *Certo* and *Nessun dubbio*. And there was Andrea who didn't want their rope. The wind blew to us the sound of his singing, this *pazzerello* flying along with the spray.

This was the last time I beheld my Andrea in full joy and health. How fine a memory! And how, by himself, he jumped up straight on to the ledge of rock and was safe and so pleased with this moment. Why, why did God have to take him so brutally? Forgive me, for I have to say this, it was truly and excessively brutal;

there was no need to be so merciless; better those sharp rocks and *finish*! Finish while he laughed and sang and the scene was noble. Better than, yes, than the terrible agonies, the long waiting, the unsuccessful operation.

I will tell you. But I must stand. I can no longer sit still and tell a story. Let me be so; let me be so. I will describe it all. It is a clear picture. I can see its every detail, and some of these details I may tell as they come, but to sit and tell this, no, I am with my memories and thoughts and with the same numbness I felt then.

There was this jump from the sea on to the rock and my friends from the lighthouse they cried 'Bravo!' And they gave me encouragement when I scolded Andrea and said, 'For God's sake, *cretino*, you put the fear of God into me!'

And he said—you must listen to what he said—'If only the sea had kept me!'

Yes, he said that. 'It would have been a wonderful death.'

And I said, 'But, Andrea, we don't want to talk of death, we want to speak of life.'

And he said, 'That's what you think.' Nothing more, nothing else . . .

We went home, climbing in that wind and the sun now setting low.

I asked myself what had changed, what had happened. Suddenly it was cold and no, not terrifying, but worse. It was like after the end of the world. And, fighting this feeling, you could only come back to those terrible words, wondering what was his deepest meaning: *If only the sea had kept me!* Andrea who loved to laugh. This, I tell you, was when I knew the real fear in me, a mysterious and terrible wondering.

179

So we went home up the mountain; after a while it was again good. He was happy and the gulls were not laughing and the sounds of the sea were far below. And the fear in me went away, like your watchdog who says to himself, now I can find my corner and sleep a little.

The next morning, the second day of August, before lunch time he said to me, 'I've a date with a girl from Materita, I'm going down again to swim with the group.' And I said, 'Good! You swim and be careful.' I did not go down myself because I had things to do in the house—not things he could do. Mending it was or darning, or something like that, perhaps washing. And he went off.

Towards evening he returned. I was already preparing the macaroni, and he came and lit the charcoal fire for me. Usually he laughed and made jokes, but now he was quiet—unusually quiet. He then said, 'I am so thirsty! I must drink something!' And he found water and he drank some water and so he was satisfied.

Soon the macaroni was ready and I put it on the table and he came to the table and ate two bites of macaroni and suddenly cried out, 'Mami! Mami! The pain! The terrible pain!'

And I could just go with him across the room to the bed and he screamed with this pain, 'For God's sake, what is the matter with my stomach? What *is* it with me?' Suddenly to have Andrea in this way, it was dreadful. I gave him a pain-killing drug and he began his first vomiting. It was a stoppage of the bowel.

Such a terrible fear came over me, but I reflected that if he too had time from his agony to feel fear, then he must be afflicted with the same kind of fear as mine, and so I tried to be calm in my manner and not to show concern. This was not easy, for I am not a one who can dissemble.

Only later I learned what the cause might have been. Down below at the lighthouse, he was with these girls and swam there. But the cause was not the sharp rocks which I feared, it was the fishermen who brought in a large fishing-boat close to the rock in order to pull it out of the sea. And he helped and, as he said, pulled very hard and in such a way that the main strain on the rope fell on him. Perhaps inside him, with the bending and pulling—how can one know? He had had an appendix operation exactly six months before we returned to Capri and perhaps there had been an intestinal lesion.

Excuse me that I cannot tell this *con calma*, too much it affects my heart. He came up and we began to eat, and then he leapt up with this terrible pain and threw himself on the bed and bashed to and fro, so unbearable was the agony. I gave him an injection which took away the pain for the moment, but later it returned.

He should have been, right at the first onset, taken to a very good clinic and operated on immediately. Instead there had to be all that evening and all that night and all the next morning. It was impossible even to engage a private boat, because the Americans, the armed forces, were still there. One could only take the passenger boat in the morning. Not even the great Cerio could have helped.

That night—you may imagine how terrible it was. He lay there, white like the sheet, moaning and twisting and half in coma and half not, and only so short a while ago he had come up from the sea, smelling of the salt of the sea and lighting for me the charcoal stove to cook our dinner.

One of my colleagues came who did not understand what was the matter. He suggested a *sitzbad* as he was perhaps thinking of a retention of urine or something, but by then I already knew it was a stoppage. To that, all he could say was '*Beh!-eh!-eh!*', shrugging his shoulders quite helpless. (A stoppage is when the intestine contorts itself round its own axis and makes a kind of knot which closes up, and of course no food can pass and above all, the circulation is strangled so that the segment in question begins to die.)

Well, I spent the night calling my poor colleague who could only repeat '*Beh!-eh!-eh!*' like a goat and say, until morning *non c'è niente da fare*. And I was thinking what can we do now for the best, to make the night move as fast as possible.

At five in the morning there was the boat. This was August the 3rd and I went with him to Naples, to the Swiss Hospital—the international hospital. We arrived and the doctor was somewhere in Naples attending a clinic. But when he came, they immediately got ready to operate, but by this time it was twelve-thirty noon. And he had to fetch another colleague for the operation, and I was outside and they called me in, and I could see that a large section of the intestine had already died off. . .

I knew immediately there was no hope. They couldn't even do a resection, which is to cut out some of the intestine and rejoin it, because it was far too late. So they sewed him up. They had to sew him up with this death in him. At the moment of opening the abdomen we all knew that his life was ended. There was no hope. Can you believe it that I felt nothing? *Nothing*! I was too finished. So now he will die, I said, and it meant nothing. Yes, I too was dying with him, as with him I had lived. Andrea was fully conscious. He was able to talk. He asked what it was. He partly understood, yes, partly he knew how serious his case was . . . That he was going to die he didn't then grasp, only that it was an extremely serious affair. During the night the operating surgeon came again but everything was hopeless, and at two in the morning he died.

It is dreadful when such a young person dies. He still had warmth and strong muscles and seemed ready to wake up. It is dreadful. A kind of astonishment as if your eyes were beholding the earth break from its balance in space and falling nowhere.

Those of the hospital notified a priest who was a Catholic. An impossible creature of a priest. He came to this twenty-year-old while he was dying; he came quite suddenly and rattled off his prayers. It was dreadful. Dreadful! I had such a shock when I thought, so *that's* your religion, *that's* how they do it here!

On this same morning of his death I had to go across with the noon boat in order to fetch money for the interment. He had after all to be buried. To go across the sea and leave him, my Andrea, dead in that white clinical room alone—how was I to have the strength to do such a thing? And it was a thing which could be done only by me, myself. I must borrow that money for the hospital, the undertakers, the funeral, the formalities, all those things.

To sit and watch him dying, even this had been not so terrible as to go away across that water, that water which then seemed like a great evil, a most detestable evil. I did not need help, nobody but Andrea himself could any more have helped. It was in a stupor the things I did, like going on the boat for Capri and walking on the decks of that boat, fast, fast; like trying to win a marathon.

I do not know what is the worst grief—that which you know you feel, or that which deprives you of all faculties. To have stayed beside my dead Andrea would have been a conscious grief, but somehow this going away from him alone and the mind quite broken and imbecile; this was too terrible, perhaps the most terrible thing.

The same face he still had in death, though now so white; the same natural smile grown into the contours of his mouth and cheeks. How may I explain that still even on that terrible boat the truth, the fact of his death, escaped me; it simply could not be possible.

Even to God I could not pray. I was too proud to pray to such a Being whom almost I could have wished to experience the same knotted agony as my innocent son. This is terrible to say, but never since then have I looked on Him for comfort, only sometimes to the Madonna who intercedes with this Deaf-Mute. But at that time, all those great omnipotent ones, I washed my hands of them, they were no good at all, and all this I told them in my silence. And so at last came Capri, and I went straight to Cerio, and I told him of the death.

On this occasion, Cerio was, as he could be, most marvellous. And very quiet, so quiet. He said, 'We do not speak of what we feel, this we know. We speak rather of what we do.' These were almost his first words. He gave me the money I needed and I went back with it to pay all and to arrange the funeral. There was a very lovely black carriage with four horses and those foolish black ostrich feathers, very Neapolitan. It went a long way through Naples to the harbour. Two of Andrea's friends, Adinolfi and Mario, had accompanied me from Capri to Naples so I shouldn't be so alone, and there we sat in this carriage behind the hearse which was like a huge black tureen with a decorated lid. They were *really* concerned and sweet, and in their eyes was the same shock as in Cerio's. They held and propped me up. I was a kind of bundle which they lugged along with them. I can only remember the beautiful black horses and the picture in my mind of Andrea laughing to be in that absurd black monument of a hearse.

I could not cry, it is not my habit, it was too terrible for that. No tears, no, not a tear. Tears are when you are released.

At the port the coffin was carried aboard and set apart. The ship's crew and many of the people knew me, and those who did not, the tourists, they all stood and they were silent in respect and in sympathy and some lowered their heads and made this honour to Andrea and to me. I have always been so grateful to all these people and some of them I was later able to thank, but the unknown ones I wished to thank them too and still wish that they had known this. So silent everybody was. It is not what you expect to see on the way to that mad place. It enabled me to pass behind the coffin as less of a bundle than I felt. I was able to put one foot before the other, and those two boys, they sustained me. At such a time you are not in this world, or in any world, you just obey some instinct. And the people, they too obeyed their instincts, they were silent and they lowered their heads. I saw this just once before we went into the cabin they had made ready.

When we arrived with the dead one on Capri, my girl

who worked for me in the surgery, my servant girl, and a few of my good friends, they cried a lot and screamed, and thus suddenly I became conscious of how frightful this all was. I just was not there, just this useless bundle.

How on earth had I managed . . .? I only left the hospital after the death in order to send the telegram to Giulietta that Andrea was dead, 'Come at once,' and when I had sent the telegram at the post office, then I knew, 'Now you don't go back to the hospital to him, but now you go to Capri, fetch the money for the funeral.' I became like a soldier when he is ordered to march one-two, one-two.

Cerio said, 'How did you manage this? You came alone, was there no one?' No, there really was no one, not even myself. I had been to Naples alone with him in all his pain, so who should have come with me now?

Then Cerio said, 'You must not return to Naples by yourself. These two, they will travel with you.' I already knew this, they had offered their services at once, at the cemetery already, where I went to see where Andrea would lie.

Cerio had told the priests that in the spirit of Andrea I didn't want a large funeral, but the most simple. All this Cerio arranged; his understanding and sympathy were wonderful at that moment. He had these gifts like a giant might, but sometimes he hid them and was so by himself that he did not even recognise you. So simple and dignified the funeral was with those simple boys, all friends of Andrea, who carried the coffin. One of them wept, so that all his face was wet as if he had dipped it in the sea.

I remember that, as I sat on a sofa in my house, all

the people from Anacapri, one after another came to tell me of their sadness and mourning; one after the other, and with great dignity, no screams, no tears. Two whole days long, people came to console me, they who had also loved Andrea and who lit candles and prayed at this time when I could not pray. Even two days after Andrea's death was too short a time for my daughter to be there, because all trains were over-full when one travelled—it was still the time of the American occupation—and so she only arrived the next day, but the grave had been left open, Cerio had arranged it, so that she could come and throw flowers on the coffin down there. Ludovico could not come because of his work, and Tutino I had not told—perhaps I had forgotten him. He came much later. Weeks later. One morning he came to my surgery. Giulietta insisted that, after the first two days, after all the people had come with the condolences, I go down to my surgery and go on doing my visits, and I obeyed her. So that is where Tutino came, and he was sad. He said, 'Why didn't you let me know?' and I believe I didn't answer him. Because I didn't talk much. I was still a bundle. And then he only said, 'I have a few photographs of Andrea which you might not have, I'll let you have them.' But he never did. I would have liked them. But what could replace Andrea? How was it possible ever to be living, to know any more joy, without Andrea?

I went on practising. And my daughter stayed. She remained for a whole year. You cannot believe her kindness. To the post she had she immediately gave notice. It was not only a consolation, it was everything. It cannot have been easy for her. But it was the only possibility, because I had been hit too hard. I would not have been capable of doing the visiting and to cook and all the household things . . . the only thing I could do was continue to give my services and run to the houses of the sick.

Ludovico and Giulietta had been wonderful children. For a while they were everything. But then there was suddenly only Andrea. He gave me that which I demanded from men, this exclusive devotion. I knew that I was everything to him and this feeling I never had with any other man. It was the accomplishment of all which I looked for in life and all which I most needed. Only thus could I use my own best gifts. Every hour of the day it was only he. The other children I did love, but it was love not enchantment. This exclusive love for Andrea came when Ludovico was twenty-five years old and Giulietta already nineteen. Andrea was fourteen. The dear God only gave me six years. But these six years I had, and they were a meaning for life and all the rest was meaningless. Here is a letter I had from him in Switzerland in April 1946, and then in August there was Capri and the sea and death.

'Mama, Mama, what a happy lovely day!

This morning I had my last examination and tonight I will know if I got through. I got to Anita's through the Langen Erlen (Long Alders), but I could not stay long with her. I asked for a piece of paper and came out here to the stream. I must now be alone. No, completely with you. I can find no words to describe the beauty of the landscape. I now sit beneath cherry trees in blossom on the banks of a babbling brook and am utterly happy. Then why do I have to write to you? Why am I so drawn to you?

You know, don't you, that I have to share all my happiness and all my sorrow with you. Whom do I have to thank after all for being so very happy today? You, only you, my mother. You gave me eyes to see all the beauty of the world, ears with which to hear this Spring-song of the birds, a heart which directs my mind to thoughts of gratitude to you, and love of nature which I can experience so fully here. Yes, my Mutterl, Switzerland *is* beautiful. Nowhere else have I seen the Spring so beautifully set out on full display as here in Switzerland. Can you remember the holidays in the Tessin? The magic of Good Friday in the chestnut tree? Wait! Now I know why above all else I have to write to you. With you I have spent the happiest hours of my life. To you belongs the happiness of today! I know how much you suffered for my sake and I shall never forget it. We are bound by a very special bond.

'You will find very few people who are as dependent on one another as you and I. I can't write any more. It is too lovely here. Have I in fact written anything? Only one more confession: that I am very, very happy and that I love you very, very much.

Your Andrea'

All women wanted him, because he was this mixture of Italian and German; passionate and yet faithful and honest. A warm and impetuous temperament, then *glücklich und traurig*. And on top of that a good-looking boy, so good-looking that once when I said this to someone she said: 'God-looking!' His nature too was God-looking and people sought him just to be happier as you may seek a fire just to be warmer. He consoled me in everything. And yet he had inside him a fearful disease. An atrophy of the brain passage. The auditory nerve was finished. He would have been deaf in ten years' time. Professor Lucker told me that in Basel. Andrea knew that he didn't hear well with one ear; he knew that he would become deaf. Perhaps he thus wished the sea should take him.

Andrea meant that kind of love which could happen only once in a lifetime. I was desperately unhappy with Tutino, and I stayed with him only because he was the father of Andrea (though perhaps he wasn't?). I always asked Tutino to return, because of Andrea. What came after he died is all shadow. Yes, I will tell you what I can of these shadows and of the sunlight which came so briefly with the second Andrea, Giulietta's son, my grandson. Here again came terrible sudden death, and with that I was finished, extinguished in every part of me.

EPILOGUE

by Graham Greene

With this last chapter the Dottoressa's memories die away. The strain of remembering proved too great. Only fragments are left, 'a broken bundle of mirrors', and one comforting dream. She dreamt that she was approaching her old house off the piazza in Caprile, and looking up she saw big Andrea on the balcony wearing a plumed hat with little Andrea beside him. He called to her to come up and she went through her door and climbed the stairs and joined them on the balcony—all this without waking. There Andrea told her that they couldn't stay as they had to go up to Monte Solaro, the mountain that looms over Caprile, but they would wave to her, he said, from there. They left her and she watched them go into the piazza and up the lane by the little restaurant, past the house where Baron von Schacht had died. Before they disappeared from sight they turned and waved to her. Only then she woke.

When I had met her first—introduced by Norman Douglas as 'the best of my two doctors, my dear. She doesn't try to stop me drinking like the other does'—nearly three years had passed since big Andrea's death. With her immense will to live she had survived that tragedy and because she could still work and was at the centre of Anacapri life she could recover time and again from her deep depressions. Nothing surely was capable any further of subduing that small square body with the big teeth ('You are a real Hun, Dottoressa'), the startlingly blue eyes, the tough electric hair as alive as a bundle of fighting snakes. She was always on the move—

down to the Marina Grande or to the Marina Piccola to have lunch with her fishermen, taking small tributes here and there, a lettuce from a stall in Caprile, an apple from the fruit shop on the Capri steps (she had delivered the *padrona*'s ninth child and thus helped her by Italian law to escape all income tax), back to the house named after the two Andreas which she loved now more than any human being. She was proud of it, the ground floor a warehouse of discarded rubbish, old mattresses and boxes, the overgrown garden where the cats and the baby were buried, proud even of the improvised douche in the bedroom made out of a tin basin and a piece of string.

Then the blows began to fall again—of which the least important were the deaths of friends. She could survive her friends as easily as she had survived the men in her life.

Norman Douglas was the first to go. He had written to me in November 1950—after warning me of the dangers of eastern travel, 'Look out for syphilis—a friend of mine came back from Malaya in a deplorable condition—I am in a pretty groggy way myself. In addition to all my other complaints I have now got erysipelas: no fun. If I can now get Babylonian itch, and a tapeworm or two, the collection will be complete. Very gloomy here. I am resting with electric light . . . fever rather high just now.'

He died at his home in the house of Kenneth Macpherson after the long pain of his incurable skin disease, unalleviated now by the visit of any boy. He had chosen death from an overdose of sleeping pills and the Dottoressa did him the last service of signing the death certificate—the nature of his death she buried as secretly as she had buried the poor girl's unwanted child in her garden. As a doctor she had no liking for the police who were the enemies of her poor and she had no respect for the letter of the law. When my maid's little boy was raped by a young man who had been deprived of sex by one of those interminable southern betrothals she left food for the criminal among the rocks of Monte Solaro where for days he hid from the *carabinieri*.

Norman Douglas's death, the death of Baron von Schacht left her only a little shaken, she would complain of loneliness more often, but she was capable in her late sixties of dancing round the tree in the piazza of Caprile from a sudden surge of fun—not because, like the rest of us, she was a little drunk. She never drank a larger measure of spirits than a doll's egg cup and her glass of wine was usually half water.

One summer I returned to Anacapri and found a great change. Andrea, her grandson, who had taken the place in her heart of the other Andrea, had been electrocuted in front of her eyes in a Zurich shoeshop just at the time when old age had forced her to give up her practice. A demanding melancholy had fallen which no friend could now alleviate for long. She was cut off from help just as Anacapri had been cut off for three days from the rest of the island by a great fire on Monte Solaro and a fall of rocks on the road from Capri. There was no comfort for her in religion. She never went to Mass. God, she repeated often, had done her too much evil. He was absurd, he was pointless, perhaps he was wicked. It was worse for her than doubting his existence. An empty universe is easier to face than a universe governed by cruelty.

I suggested these memoirs to her because I thought they might provide a sort of therapy, but the therapy was to prove too dangerous. Through someone's indiscretion her son was enabled to hear some of the tapes. He was no longer the little Ludovico of whom she had spoken so tenderly. He was the father of a family. He was successful. He was one of the heads of the Swiss tourist industry. Above all—it was her worst reproach—he had become Swiss to the core. He was shocked at the very idea of publication and he spoke to her so harshly that in her fear and rage she had her first stroke. Her eyes began rapidly to fail, and she had loved reading only next to work. Now that was being taken from her. All the same, though she had quarrelled with her son, she loved him dearly, and then suddenly even he died.

I had been accustomed to say jokingly when she complained of all her aches and pains and went into lurid descriptions—usually at meal times—of the dark happenings in her bowels, 'Dottoressa, you will survive us all.' It was proving true, but there was no happiness for her in that. Only very seldom now the old cracking laugh, so similar to Norman's, rang out at one of the early memories her son had found so scandalous.

For one like myself who for twenty-eight years has passed some part of every year in Anacapri there is a strong sense of emptiness there today. Dottoressa Moor had been indeed an impossible woman. Selfish to all except her patients (to them a bit of a bully), egotistical, self-pitying often, she could drain her friends dry for the sake of her own survival—I once had to fly to Ravello to escape those Promethean curses against the God who had tied her to a rock of suffering. Yet one forgave her everything, and Caprile and Anacapri today seem to have lost their centre without her. Three times a day in the long street I am stopped for news of the Dottoressa and there is no news to give except that she still survives, her house sold, an exile in the Switzerland she has never loved. Half-blind she could no longer live alone. During her last year on Capri she had spent forty-eight hours in a coma on her bed before she was found, wet through with vomit, by her daily woman.

For forty years the peasants had come to her, and the fishermen, to have their pulses taken in the street, or in her house to have their blood pressure measured, and she would say to them, 'Everything is in order. Could also be better. Don't drink so much and eat less salt,' and next day the patients would bring a fee in the form of a fish, some salad or fruit, a sweet cake, sometimes a bottle of wine which would last her for weeks. They trusted no other doctor, and I don't know who now has taken her place. I was with her when she left the island for the last time. Gracie Fields came and sang to her beside the taxi waiting in the square of Caprile by the steps which went down to her old house, which was fast becoming like the ruin she had bought, and her last embrace and last tears were for a fishwife in the port. Even at the final moment when the gangplank of the *aliscafo* was lowered I was afraid she might turn and run from us up and up the cliff path and into the shelter of the house as she had run forty years back from the peasants with cudgels.

There was a song the Dottoressa remembered from her childhood. It wasn't the song Gracie Fields sang.

And when I have sold my house,
And have drunk all the lolly,
Then my father says:
I was a soldier, who drank it all.

Where does one end up, with the drink?
Where does one end up, with the drink?
In heaven,
Where Peter will be,
Who'll pour us a slivovitz,
Who'll pour us a slivovitz.

Who'll be at my funeral?
Who'll be at my funeral?
The dishes, and knives and forks,
The wine and the beer,
And the pub-keeper's wife will crawl along with me,
And the pub-keeper's wife will crawl along with me.

And who will sweep the streets for us now?
And who will sweep the streets for us now?
The most honourable gentlemen,
With the golden star,
They'll sweep the streets for us then.

Yet before she was finally beaten down by the death of little Andrea she had possessed even in her seventies a quality of passionate living which I have known in no other woman, though I tried to give it another form and habitation in Aunt Augusta of *Travels with my Aunt*.

I remember one evening when we went together to a film about Attila in the Anacapri cinema and how that whole night she couldn't sleep a wink for the images which raced through her mind of Anthony Quinn making his wars and his rapes. I had been right in telling her that she had the teeth of a Hun. So too after a performance of *Tristan and Isolde* at the Vienna opera she spent a sleepless night with the erotic music repeating in her head. She had lost her last lover as she was approaching seventy, but the passion of sex was always ready to wake.

Once she made a list of the men who had played however small a part in her life. Here it is carefully numbered in chronological order and headed simply 'Men'. It doesn't always quite coincide with the memories, but perhaps there were too many of them to remember all clearly.

MEN

(1) When I was seven years old, there was a waiter down in the Prater who caressed me pretty firmly wherever he could get hold of me.

(2) In the Einsiedlergasse there was a stable. There was a stableboy who I liked a lot. I can no longer remember what happened. I was nine years old.

(3) One summer in Lainz, there was a cousin, the son of my mother's sister from Germany. We were the same age, around ten, and wanted to try it, so we hid in a little wood. There were jasmin bushes. We were only curious, it was a load of fun, and we were playing at something amusing. We had no feelings. The grown-ups noticed something and didn't let us out into the garden any more.

(4) When I went to primary school, there was a chemist's shop near the Neville Bridge in the Fifth District. The druggist took me behind the counter. I was in mourning clothes, because my great-uncle had died. The druggist was a fat, ugly chap, he wanted to take my pants down. I didn't say anything at home because I was afraid.

(5) Our cook, the Hungarian Resi, wanted to fiddle around, and when I wouldn't do her bidding, she beat me. Once she beat me so hard in the bathroom that I had a crooked back. I was ten years old at the time.

(6) On the third floor of our house there was a businessman. I had to sit on his knee. I sat, I was kissed and I was given sweets.

(7) In St Wolfgang there were the two Pater boys, Paul and Max. I liked Max. Paul was bigger and we mucked about and he deflowered me. I was scared but nothing happened.

(8) In St Wolfgang the landlord messed around.

(9) I went to the Language School Weiser, I was fourteen, my friend was Frieda Abeles, whose cousin was Max Adler. He was fifteen and he went to technical school. He was the first real one with birth control and all that. And Abeles split on us.

His appearance: medium tall, dark brown, pleasant voice, gay, friendly face, lovely eyes, good walk, he was full of precision and hope. Nice, intelligent and sensible. Laughed a lot. My parents thought: childhood sweethearts.

(10) In Grossgmain, I met a young Belgian on the tennis court. I was fifteen or sixteen. We made trips up the Lofererberg from Reichenhall. He was the right one, for two or three weeks. He was around twenty-five then.

(11) Dornfeld was a lawyer. I helped him with his Roman law. In the same house was the Belgian, but Dornfeld was a very short thing, perhaps there even was nothing with him.

(12) In Millstadt, at the tennis tournament there was Szenes, I think an Hungarian, seventeen years old, with whom I went mountaineering and so on . . .

(13) Norbert Baudisch did his matura in Salzburg. I went with him to Florence, and lived in the Pensione Daddi.

(14) At some point I went alone to Rome, and in the Cafe Greco I met Tolleg. He was a small Frenchman, who drew. I dragged Tolleg back to Vienna and also to Mama. She must have been a very innocent woman.

(15) Georg Schalinger was a colleague from medical school. Such a gay funny red-haired one.

(16) When the comet was there, there was another medical student colleague, an Italian, Leonardo. With him we went to the Hermannskogel. I preferred him to all the others.

(17) Doctor Munt was an assistant, a medical

assistant, a mild Pole, very melancholy, took everything seriously, and even wanted to marry me.
And that's why I finished with him very quickly.

(18) Alfi Gabriel.

(19) Gigi Moor.

(20) There was this Bedouin in Gafsa, but it was
as good as nothing.

(21) In Seelisberg in Switzerland, there was the
Russian tenor Wolkow.

(22) Beniamino Tutino.

(23) A sailor in Naples. That was at the time of
Tutino in Positano. I no longer liked Tutino. On
the ship from Sorrento to Naples there was a
sailor. We went to the Hotel Metropole in the harbour. He couldn't pay for the room and I also had
no money. I left my wedding ring as surety, and
later collected it again. The man later went to
America.

(24) I once went to visit my mother in Vienna and
she had a lodger, but he was an idiot.

(25) On the beach of Serapis in Gaeta there was an
Italian, but, if I remember rightly, he only kissed
or something.

(26) The flying officer in Rome, who was perhaps
Andrea's father.
Then for a while, nothing, and then a few things.

(27) Desiderio in Capri.

(28) Brunetti, the teacher also in Capri.

(29) The pharmacist.

(30) Edwin Cerio.
Between 1939 and 1946, in Switzerland, I only
looked after Andrea.

(31) Now, a few years ago, there was a peasant in Anacapri. He wanted to marry me, and he had a very lovely garden, that I must say for him . . . But I didn't want to.

(32) Julius Kmachl was in the Mozarteum in Salzburg. He already wanted to marry me between the wars and later also. It was a long story. He was tall, had wavy hair, was cultivated, musical, but he was not attractive to me. He was fond of me, but I didn't want to. (Of course there was a bit of an affair.)

When she had made this list, she added a short piece which she called 'Men in General'.

'The best relationship was always friendship. To have someone who loved one. The erotic is part of this, and that I understood. Passion I only had with Tutino. Love is more durable, stronger, and encompasses much more. Passion is present. One is capable of hating the man at the same time.

'The thing with Tutino would never have happened, if I hadn't just been recovering from a three months' bout of typhoid. I was full of the desire to live after it.

'Gigi was wild. He locked me out, and the children cried inside the house. Both the men avoided each other. When Gigi became hot tempered, it was dreadful. He became chalk-white, like the bleached wall. And with that his eyes would blaze! When he was not drunk, the sudden temper was even worse. His parents were terrified when he joined the army. He had something morbid about him. He was wrong to go away. He cried at my mother's. There were weeping scenes. Why did he never come back? He always had others.

'With Tutino I was around thirty-five to forty years old. With Tutino, it was a mania, a thing bewitched, I never really did it with my brain. But I always did that which I wanted to do.

'My mother once wanted to tell me the facts of life: I was never to kiss a man, I was not to let him touch me, nor to go with him alone into a room. But I only let my mother subjugate me once, when she plaited my three plaits, and then there was a tugging. By that time I had long since been with Paul Pater in the dependence of the hotel.

'Women are lying things. One has to drag them by the hair, as I did with my only girl-friend, with Frieda. I was never sorry for her for a single moment. I would like to live in a state of men only. Women should be eradicated.'

My favourite memory of her was of once when she came to London and I played to her on my gramophone Kurt Weill's setting of Brecht's song '*Wie Man Sich Bettet*' (As You Make Your Bed). She listened with her thick legs apart like a Henry Moore figure. 'That is right, that is so . . .' Three times I had to play the record, while she listened with her blue eyes alight and her great teeth bared.

For, as you make your bed so must you lie,
There's nobody to cover you up there,
If somebody's to do the stepping, it will be me,
If somebody's to be stepped on, it will be you.

She had made a good many beds and she had done a good deal of stepping. There were moments in her broken and expressive English when she touched poetry as when she spoke of her bad year 1964, 'When the cold of the world around us began to be unbearable,' and surely the account of Andrea's death deserves a permanent place in literature. She could make a character live a short vivid life like someone in a story of Boccaccio, in her moments of bawdry she resembled the Wife of Bath, and when she was happy and rambling over her sexual memories I was often reminded of Mrs Bloom's monologue, 'and yes I said yes I will Yes.' The past to her was never dead. Once after dinner in Vienna I hunted out with her the little hotel near the railway which she had visited with the actor Hoffmann. It was still standing after bombardment and occupation, but she refused to go in for fear that the night porter might recognise the young girl who had come to make love there sixty years before.

*

On February 23 1975 the Dottoressa died, in exile, in the Switzerland she had never loved. She was in her 90th year. She had felt some pride in the slow growth of her book, though she never really believed it would be published, and she was able to hold a proof copy in her hands for a few days before she died. At the end her Promethean spirit was quiet. The President of the Immortals had finished his game with her.